CHE-MOMENT

BEST WISHES
ON YOUR JOURNEY
THROUGH LIFE !

WITH LOVE,

CHE-MOMENT

Life Lessons, Facing Death, and Surviving Cancer (AML M2) Leukemia and beyond. A Medical Rep's story of how FAITH, POSITIVE ATTITUDE, and EXERCISE can beat the odds.

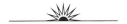

Chris J. Hamilton

authorHOUSE®

AuthorHouse™
1663 Liberty Drive
Bloomington, IN 47403
www.authorhouse.com
Phone: 1-800-839-8640

Published by AuthorHouse   06/13/2013

ISBN: 978-1-4817-6245-8 (sc)
ISBN: 978-1-4817-6244-1 (hc)
ISBN: 978-1-4817-6246-5 (e)

Library of Congress Control Number: 2013910534

CONTENTS

ACKNOWLEDGEMENTS ix

PROLOGUE. xiii

CHAPTER 1. 1
GROWING UP, FAMILY, AND MY FIRST GUARDIAN
ANGEL EXPERIENCE

CHAPTER 2. 8
SUCCESSES, MONEY, AND AWARDS DO NOT MEAN
ANYTHING

CHAPTER 3. 16
BACK TO HOW MY JOURNEY BEGAN

CHAPTER 4. 20
11/11/11 AND HOW MY LIFE TOOK A TURN

CHAPTER 5. 25
MO-HAWK AND READY TO TAKE ON THE FIGHT/
JOURNEY

CHAPTER 6. 35
DO NOT SWEAT THE SMALL STUFF—
DARK DAYS AND BAD NEWS

CHAPTER 7. 43
WHY ARE THERE NOT ANY PICTURES OF AML
SURVIVORS IN THE UNC CANCER LOBBY

CHAPTER 8. 48
PLAN B, BIG DECISIONS, AND LAST RIGHTS

CHAPTER 9 . . . . **58**
STEM CELL TRANSPLANT AND MY NEW BIRTHDAY

CHAPTER 10 . . . . **71**
MY CLOSING DAYS ON THE BONE MARROW
TRANSPLANT FLOOR

CHAPTER 11 . . . . **76**
SECU HOUSE AND POST-TRANSPLANT CARE

CHAPTER 12 . . . . **90**
ANOTHER SURPRISE, ANOTHER GUARDIAN ANGEL
EXPERIENCE, AND MY NEW LIFE

CHAPTER 13 . . . . **96**
EXAMPLES OF MY CAREPAGES/BLOGS

CHAPTER 14 . . . . **113**
EPILOGUE, TAKEAWAYS, AND PICTURES

DEFINITIONS AND MEDICAL
TERMINOLOGY SECTION **131**

A Portion of the Profits For Each Book Sold will go to:

* The Bone Marrow Foundation in New York, NY

* The Cancer Care Fund with The Foundation of First Health in Pinehurst, NC

* UNC Lineberger Cancer Hospital Patients Fund in Chapel Hill, NC

* National Marrow Donor Program in Minneapolis, MN

ACKNOWLEDGEMENTS

This book was written with special thanks to following people because without the Love and Support I received during my journey, I definitely could have had a different outcome. As you read through these acknowledgements, please take the time to pick up the phone and call someone that may need you during his/her personal battle. As you read my book there will be mentions and specific thank you's to describe more what these people meant to me.

I would like to thank the following people and organizations in no particular order and I hope to God I do not forget anybody:

* Billy Hamilton Roehm (Brother), thank you from the bottom of my heart. Your stem cells saved my life. I love you forever and ever!
* Joseph Roehm, thank you for you spiritual guidance and your never ending faith in miracles. I love you!
* Madeleine Hamilton (Mom), thank you for staying by my side during my transplant; you are my Eagle and I love you so much for all that you have done in my lifetime.
* William Hamilton (Dad), thank you for your love, support, and guidance during my two years and always being there for Billy and me when we needed you.
* Laura Hamilton (Spouse), thank you for being my caregiver for two years—I know it was tough emotionally and sometimes a thankless job. I could not have done it without you. Thank you so much!
* Riley Hamilton (Oldest Son) and Brennan Hamilton (Youngest Son), you two were my inspiration through it all. I will always Love both of you to God's house and back. Thank you for keeping your grades up and being MEN during my two years.
* Dan Matthews PA-C, thank you for your great care of my medical needs and your friendship through the years. We sure have had some great laughs!
* Seven Lakes Family Care Nurses and Staff
* Stewart and Donna Winterson, thank you for being my biggest cheerleaders.

* Elizabeth Kerr, thank you for the prayers, holy water and St. Pio's special items.
* Mark Foley, thank you for your caring and support during this last year.
* Ken and Kathy Smith (In-laws), thank you for your love, support and all that darn good food that Adam and I ate during our three months at the SECU House.
* Adam Smith (Brother-in-law), thank you for devoting over two months of your time, love, and patience with being my caregiver at the SECU House.
* Aunt Palma, thank you for holding two Healing Masses with Father Domingo.
* UNC Lineberger Comprehensive Cancer Hospital
* UNC 4-Onc Nurses
* Karen Mitchell and Natasha Hanks, thank you for being the first smiling faces I see at The Bone Marrow Transplant Clinic. You two are a blast.
* UNC Bone Marrow Unit Nurses
* UNC Bone Marrow Clinic
* UNC Lineberger Comprehensive Cancer Hospital Doctors
* UNC Food Services, Thank you Allegra for making me feel welcomed.
* Moore Regional Cancer Center, Pinehurst, NC
* Moore Regional Radiation Oncology Nurses and Doctors
* Moore Regional Outpatient Cancer Center Nurses and Doctors
* Moore Regional Outpatient Cancer and Transfusion Center Nurses
* Yale New Haven Cancer Hospital Doctors and Nurses
* Fayetteville Otolaryngology Doctors and Nurses
* Cape Fear Valley Hospital and Cancer Center
* Bone Marrow Foundation, New York, NY
* Jason and Annie Smith, thank you for your friendship and the fly fishing Jason.
* SECU House Staff and Foundation, Chapel Hill, NC thank you for being there.
* Father, Ricardo F. Sanchez, thank you for your guidance—I do believe in miracles.
* Anne and Joe Scirrino, thank you for all the great Italian food and your friendship.

* Lula Poulos, Lula's Cafe in Southern Pines for your kind heart and great food.
* Aaron Gootman, thank you for your support, books, and friendship.
* Joan Roth, thank you for your guidance and faith in miracles—you are an Angel.
* Yvonne McEvoy thank you for the poem and pineapple chocolates. Love you!
* Dina Donohue, thank you for the edibles. Love the pineapple chocolates and you!
* Dan Bruder, thank you for your friendship and heartfelt write-up on Facebook.
* Steve and Kay Miller, thank you for all of your help with the kids and your friendship.
* Lauren Shampo, thank you for being the first eyes with book and for your great ideas and friendship over the years.
* Sal DeFilippo, thank you for your support with web pages, promotions and your friendship over the years.
* The Owl's Nest, thank you for all of your support and FAU goodies.
* Kappa and Greg Muldoon, thank you for all the FAU gear and support.
* Todd and Moreen Mead, thank you for allowing me to stay in your rental house for five days, so that I would not contaminate my family with radiation.
* Charles and Erin Fasanati, for the Giordano's Pizza, special knitted blanket and love and support. You two have been so giving and loving—thank you!
* Ken McBean, thank you for visiting and giving hockey tickets to my boys during my journey. They had a blast and it definitely took their minds off of reality.
* Harry Cross, thank you for your friendship and for kicking me in the butt to go see my ENT. Thank you for the hockey tickets.
* Dan Grose, thank you for visiting me during my journey. You most definitely lifted my spirits.

Thanks also to the following people for your love and support:

* Patience and Tom Burns, Brenda McMullen, Kurt Dionne, Asheley and Scott Underwood, Bill Nichols, Paul Jones, Ken McBean, Amy Borman, Francis Wells, Pete Zubay, Harry Cross, The McNamara's, Dan Brennan, Lisa Sheehan, Ken and Laura Begnoche, Perry Kemp, Freddy Lange, Tracy Medlin, Daryl Edwards, Ed and Lana Schempp, Mike Stephens, Dr. Wayne and Louise Lucas, Laura Creeden, and Dr. Wayne Hatfield.

More thanks and pictures at the end of book with many more useful tips to help with your success.

PROLOGUE

We all have key moments in our lives that serve as wake-up calls or warning signs that our life is on the wrong path. One of my *CHE-MOments* in life was the day I looked back on my journey and realized that my cancers were all signs that my life had spun out of control. I focused on many of the wrong aspects of life. I worried about all the small stuff instead of enjoying the big picture and what life had to offer.

This book was written to serve as a survival guide for beating cancer/ other devastating diseases; moreover, to serve as a reminder that living life is more valuable than cruising through focusing on all the wrong things. This book is also dedicated to everyone that has been touched by cancer, to everyone that is fighting cancer, and to everyone that lost a battle to cancer. I am a survivor of four cancers including AML (Acute Myelogenous Leukemia) M2 with a three-way translocation. My journey has been two years, and there is no doubt that my battle is in my rearview mirror today.

I, like many people, was caught-up in what I thought was relevant; money, success, President's Club sales awards, material possessions, etc. I was ignoring my health. Moreover, I was not recognizing the warning signs that something was terribly wrong. Trust me, when one realizes that there is a higher calling or more important focus in life; one can finally live and enjoy what life has to offer.

I hope this book inspires you to keep your head up during your journey/ fight. I also want you to know that there is always someone else out there that has it worse than you and I. You will get many survival tips throughout my book that will help you navigate through your journey and shed more light on the stem cell transplant process. You will also have a roadmap or a summary of what to expect with leukemia, MDS, throat cancer, thyroid cancer, etc. I hope you enjoy my book and come away with many life lessons, as well as many survival tools.

I have made this book a fast and easy read, so that those going through chemo treatments can get through the book. I have also included a medical terminology and definitions section in the back of the book to make this a one-stop read. If you run into a medical term that you do not understand, please pause and look it up in the back of the book. This book also has many other life lessons and surprises along the way which I promise will hold your interest, including guardian angels and near death experiences. I also promise that you will get something from my experience that will help you understand cancer. Further, I intentionally left out many details and painful experiences because a two-year journey could take up to 1,000 pages.

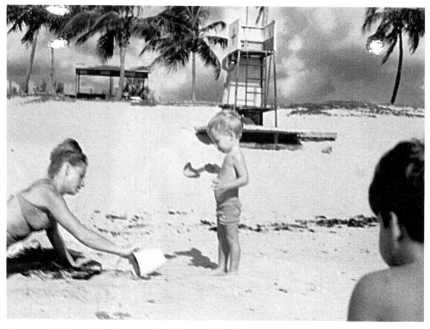

Picture of Mom Hamilton with Billy and I at Boynton Beach, Florida. I am holding the shovel, while (Brother) Billy was setting up the castle. Love you both so much!!

CHAPTER 1

GROWING UP, FAMILY, AND MY FIRST GUARDIAN ANGEL EXPERIENCE

Chapel Hill, North Carolina—11/11/11

Reality slapped me in the face like Don Corleone in *The Godfather* slaps Johnny Fontaine and says; "You can act like a man—what's the matter with you?" I just found out that I was diagnosed with Acute Myelogenous Leukemia (AML) at 4:00pm on Friday November 11, 2011. I just completed two surgeries to remove squamous cell carcinoma of the left tonsil and papillary carcinoma of the left and right thyroid.

The flurry of news hit me dead in the chest! I was freaking out and felt like my world just collapsed. I mean come on—I just finished fighting cancer for eight months and thought that my battle was complete. Do I have enough in the tank to battle AML and a stem cell transplant? AML can take up to two years to cure, and the odds for survival are devastatingly low. So, the only thing I could do was act like a man and make the best of my situation. My story will soon unfold before you.

"And in the end it's not the years in your life that count; it's the life in your years."

This quotation by Abraham Lincoln is an important quotation to think about or at least it was for me. If you take anything away from this book, please live life the best you can no matter what you are going through currently. Please make every day count from this day forward.

I was born and raised in Boynton Beach, Florida. My Father, Bill Hamilton was born in Rye, New York and worked as a police officer in Boynton Beach. He worked hard and moved up to Chief of Police. It was always tough being the son of a police officer, because Dad always knew what I was up to every minute of the day. If I was ever in trouble, my Father knew it before I even walked through the door.

My Mother, Madeleine Hamilton was born in Holland and grew up in Ipswich, Massachusetts. She moved south and met my Father at Seacrest High School in Delray Beach, Florida. Mom caught his eye during one of his shifts as a school crossing guard. They have been happily married for 50 plus years.

My brother Billy is four years my senior and my only sibling. Billy would prove to save my life from AML and MDS with his stem cells. Billy and I were always up to no good as children, and he was always daring me to do things growing up. He and I were also constantly dreaming of being medical professionals. That dream would be the start of my future in medical sales; moreover, my education would play a major role in my surviving 25% odds of beating my cancers.

I grew up a happy, active, and fun-loving child. I enjoyed surfing, soccer, football, fishing, running track, and of course wreaking havoc with my brother Billy. I attended school at Delray Elementary, Barton Elementary, Lantana Junior High School, and Santaluces High School; all located in Palm Beach County. I was a hard working kid and always found odd jobs around the neighborhood.

I will never forget a life lesson that my Father taught me back when I was 13 years old. Back in the late 1970s to early 1980s, the new craze was Nike shoes. I just had to have a pair of these magnificent shoes that many kids were wearing in school. My Father worked as a police officer, and we could not afford the luxuries that were afforded by many. I also wanted the new AC/DC album *Back in Black*.

Dad said to me, "Son you need to go earn some money to buy those expensive Nike shoes. They are out of their mind on how expensive they are." Dad was always teaching me life lessons and street smarts.

Well, I listened to my Dad. I rode my bike to the end of my street where a plant farm was located. I was determined to get my shoes quickly so that

I could enjoy them. I knocked on the door of trailer located on the plant farm and asked for the owner. I introduced myself and asked him if he needed any help with loading plants on their trucks.

The owner was thrilled and offered me a job right there on the spot. I asked how much he paid and he answered that he only could afford a couple of bucks per hour. I was thrilled and told him that I could work every weekend and after school if needed.

The first weekend I worked 12 hours, and this was tough work. I had to load semi trucks up with plants all day long. At the end of the day, I was tired, and covered in soil from head to toe. By the third weekend, I had enough to buy my Nike shoes, a *Led Zeppelin* album, and the *AC/DC* album. What a vast sense of accomplishment I felt that day. My Father was truly proud that I figured out a way to get my shoes and albums I wanted. Thank you Dad for instilling the knowledge of what hard work can get a person in life. I am not sure he appreciated the rock-n-roll blasting from the back of the house though.

Another great lesson that my father taught me was how important a college education was back then. I will never forget this life lesson because it did not take me long to figure out that he was right. I had just turned 18 and graduated high school from Santaluces High in Lantana, Florida. Most of my friends were already attending college, and I was not ready for more school.

My father suggested that I work with my neighbor Charlie Cale. Charlie owned a successful construction company and was always in the need of good help. I met with Charlie, and he was more than happy to hire me. Charlie headed out every morning at 5:30am, and he reminded me to pack a lunch. I was excited to work with Charlie because he was a character. He was particularly charismatic and always had exceptional jokes, not to mention his wife Nancy was a prominent cook.

Boy 5:30am sure did come early on the first day! During my first hour on the job, Charlie gave me the responsibility of running the cement mixer. My body and clothes were covered in white powder. Once the cement was ready, I had to pour it into a wheelbarrow and push it through fine sand.

The sand was ankle deep and felt more like quick sand. What did I get myself into?

The construction crew was using the cement quicker than I could make it, and they were yelling at me all day to get it to them faster. I felt like Lucile Ball on the famous chocolate scene on *I love Lucy*. I just could not keep up. I also had to balance the wheelbarrow, and push it up planks of wood to reach the building that we were constructing. We took a short break to eat lunch, although it was not like the movies where the construction crew sits around and whistles at female passersby.

When I returned home, my Father asked me, "what the heck happened to you?" Just by his tone, I knew that he and Charlie were in cahoots. I woke up the next day, barely getting out of bed; I felt as if I was pummeled by a professional boxer. I managed to pull myself up yet again for another day of abuse. Charlie greeted me that morning and said, "how are you feeling?" I replied great! We arrived at the construction site just as the sun was rising.

Charlie put me on the cement mixer again. As I worked throughout the day, I kept asking myself; do you want to do this crap for the rest of your life? Well, I lasted two weeks, and then I sat down with my Father. I told him that I was aware of what he was trying to teach me, and that it convinced me that I needed to apply for college that day. He laughed and said, "Son, I am so proud of you."

See my Father has a master's degree from Pepperdine University in Malibu, California. I tell him that he has a master's degree from the school of hard knocks, and he always chuckles. He is tough to outsmart and has always been a fabulous father figure. Thanks again Dad for instilling that work ethic that has helped me so much in my lifetime.

Please, do not get me wrong; my Mother Madeleine was, and is the best mother anyone could ever have. She dedicated her life to Billy and me by staying home with us until I was 18. She taught me how to be humble. She taught me to always use my manners and, most of all, to treat people exactly how I wanted to be treated. Mom was always as cool as a cucumber and as happy as a lark. Everyone always said that I had the sweetest and most giving mother. I could not agree more.

Mom was always there for all of us and always put her family first. I will never forget her loading all of my friends up countless times, with all of our surfboards tied down to the roof of her car. She would drive us up coast to Hobe Sound, Florida every time the north swells would kick up. She sat for countless hours watching us surf, and she also collected driftwood for her garden at home.

Thank you Mom for your endless love, unselfishness, and sense of humor. Furthermore, thank you for your support throughout my first 45 years, and most of all for being my Eagle. You also give hope to everyone that you meet, and you are the most giving person I know.

During college, I parked cars at the Breakers Hotel in Palm Beach, Florida. I also worked at other great employers such as The Boca Raton Resort and Club as a bellhop. I met many famous people while working at the Breakers and Boca Raton Resort; including, Princess Diana, Prince Charles, President Ronald Reagan, First Lady Nancy Reagan, Dan Marino, Madonna, Robin Williams, Chevy Chase, Steven Tyler, George Burns, and many more. Both hotels were built back in the 1920s and have years of history behind them. Boy, I sure was lucky to have those jobs in college.

One more story about my childhood. I had mentioned in the chapter title that I had a run-in with my guardian angel. One beautiful morning in Boynton Beach, Billy and I went on a bike ride. He and I were always on the go, and we enjoyed growing up in a small town.

We were on our way up to Bethesda Memorial Hospital, where we loved to drive our bikes routinely. Billy and I ran into some trouble or should I say trouble ran into me. An elderly man was speeding and did not see me on my bike. Before my Brother and I could react, the man blew through the stop sign, and struck me on my bike.

Like a runaway train without a conductor, he did not realize that I was stuck under the car or that he even hit something. Those that live in South Florida understand and see this often with the elderly population. He traveled a couple of blocks with me pinned under the car until someone waved him to a stop. All I remembered was being able to ride in the

Ambulance, which to a young boy was a big deal. The doctors could not believe it. I walked away with only a small scratch.

How was this possible? How did I not get crushed under his car? My Father went back to the scene of the accident, and he found a couple of long lines dug out in the pavement. This was from my pedal and my handle bars being pushed into the asphalt. My bike was a total loss and crushed beyond recognition.

How did I survive such an unexplainable accident? How did I not have several broken bones? My only explanation was that this was my first brush with a miracle and would prove to me that guardian angles do exist. Who protected me that day? Over the years, like most people, I have questioned spirituality and if there is life after life? I have definitely opened my eyes to believing more after this bike accident.

A great quotation that comes to mind when I think of guardian angels:
"People only see what they are prepared to see."
—Ralph Waldo Emerson

Do you believe in miracles? Do you believe in guardian angels? After that bike accident, I am a believer. There is no way anyone can just walk away from an accident like mine without an injury. We never know when it is our moment to have our time card punched, and only one higher being knows when that time is. As you will read, I think you will agree that my time on earth is not over until my mission is complete. See, time is all we got, and some of us find out that we have less time than we thought we had. You must also keep hope and know that we can survive almost anything with prayer and positive thinking; I am 100% certain that this is true.

My mission is to ultimately reach as many cancer/AML and MDS patients as possible and give them hope through this book. I started writing this book because the nurses and friends that took care of me told me that I should do so. They constantly asked me how I kept my head up during the entire two year journey. I will touch upon how this is possible throughout the book and hope that I can make a difference in your life.

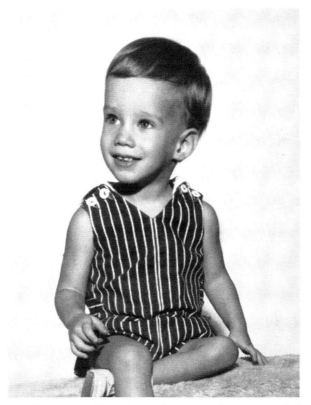

Here is a picture from my childhood, proudly wearing homemade clothing that my Mother Madeleine made for me. Thank you for your love and support Mom and Dad. Billy and I truly appreciate everything you have done for us over the years.

CHAPTER 2

SUCCESSES, MONEY, AND AWARDS DO NOT MEAN ANYTHING

Another great quotation that helped me understand that I ignored my health in order to become successful. **"Judge your success by what you had to give up in order to get it."** The Dalai Lama XIV

The Dalai Lama XIV nailed this quotation right on the head. Do you know anyone that is giving up their health to obtain success in life? Think long and hard about what causes people stress because it just might be that stress that consumes them or causes illness. I definitely feel that stress was a contributing factor in my life and with my cancers.

After graduating college in 1991 with my Bachelor's in Business Administration from Florida Atlantic University (FAU). I continued on into the workforce. I met my wonderful spouse Laura just as I was graduating college, and this is who gave me my two beautiful Sons.

Riley and Brennan, now 16 and 13 years old, are and will always be the center of my life. Oh the joy of children, especially when they are such fabulous men as mine. I cannot explain how strong and understanding they have been through my journey. Nothing wavered! Their grades, their attitudes, their zest for life, their sports; I mean nothing gave. They were my inspiration. Riley loves playing hockey, and Brennan loves playing soccer. They have been playing since they were four years old, and I have had the pleasure of coaching them in many sports including football, hockey, and soccer.

My dream was to work for Johnson & Johnson (J&J) coming out of college, and I knew that it would be a tough goal to accomplish. I always wanted to work in medical sales and work with medical professionals. I tried contacting and interviewing with J&J, and I received the proverbial door in the face each time. I did, nonetheless, receive great advice at the interviews. I was told that I should get as much sales training and experience as I could obtain. I was also told that I should strive to be in the top 2 to 5% in sales no matter where I worked.

I worked for a few Fortune 500 companies including Spectracide, The Glidden Company and Ralph Lauren Paints. I received several President's Cup awards throughout my tenure, and I was always in the top 5% in sales. I was also awarded the number one sales rep in the nation a couple of times with Spectracide. My final position at The Glidden Company was a regional manager position in which I was responsible for $30,000,000 in sales and 14 sales representatives. My region was Mid-Atlantic and included South Carolina, North Carolina, Virginia, and District of Columbia. This regional manager position was what relocated my family to Cary, North Carolina.

Knowing that I finally bolstered my resume, it was time to go after my dream. I had an interview scheduled just before a family vacation in October of 2004. I knew this was my best chance to get hired, and I made sure that I was prepared. I prepared a brag book which showed all of my sales accomplishments, and I had proof of all my awards and President's Cups. I will never forget the interview, because it was with a district manager with whom I would spend many years with at two different companies.

The interview also included another district manager and the regional manager. The interview reminded me of a firing squad; asking questions at a rapid pace. However, it went well. Have you ever walked into an interview and felt that everything was aligned for you? This interview felt that way to me. The hiring process was about two months long and included second, third, and fourth interviews. The hiring process also included psychological testing and background check. I finally received my answer on December 11, 2004. My new manager called me, and I started my career with J&J on December 27, 2004. Wow, I remember being elated, and I called my family to start the celebration. That news definitely made our family vacation a blast.

This job would serve as a base not only for my family but also for my education in the medical field. The training at J&J is by far the best in the medical industry. My original job with J&J was in the pharmaceutical division. The medications that I sold were Levaquin, Aciphex, and Ultram. The training was intense and learning the antibiotic market was particularly tough. Just studying the pathogens and where they cause inflammation and infections was mind boggling. Heck, even pronouncing the pathogens was difficult for a boy from Boynton Beach.

Just pronouncing streptococcus pneumoniae, enunciated as strep-to-coc-cus na-moan-eye-a, and recalling what organs can be affected with inflammation from this pathogen or bacteria was difficult. We in the industry referred to this pathogen as strep pneumo because it was to hard to discuss using its actual scientific name. I still remember to this day that Levaquin was 99.9% effective in killing strep pneumo; which is the most common pathogen that causes infections of the sinuses and lungs. I was especially lucky to have Levaquin in my bag. I also remember all the disease states, also known as indications, that Levaquin treated and the proper dosages for each indication. The scary thing is that I have not sold Levaquin in over five years!

During my first year with J&J I was fortunate enough to receive many awards and accolades. I was named Rookie of the Year in 2005, and my working partner Lauren and I ended up being in the top three representatives in the nation for 2005. There were over 1,500 sales representatives in the primary care sales force nationwide. Not only did we make President's Cup in 2005, Lauren and I also received a trip to Japan for being in the top 1% in Levaquin sales. Our President's Cup celebration was in Cabo San Lucas, Mexico. Cabo was definitely one of the best trips Laura and I ever experienced.

My next stop with J&J was with Ethicon Endo-Surgery and was a significant move up in the J&J world. J&J has 250 companies within their umbrella and this was one of the top companies they were fortunate enough to have. This training was bar none the best and was almost three months long. As a surgical rep, people are trained in many facets of the medical industry. Ethicon went as far as allowing us many days of actual surgery on live porcine/hogs. This way we could explain in detail how to use the many products during surgeries. My main product was *Harmonic Technology*, which was a device that had two blades that moved together 55,000 times per second. The heat produced by the rapid motion caused *Harmonic* to cut while simultaneously sealing the tissue. There was little to no collateral damage to other tissue. I also was trained on almost 200 other products or instruments used during surgery. The training day started at 7:00am with an exam every morning on what we had learned the prior day and night. I often went to bed at 2:00am because of the intense studying.

This training was well worth it, and would help me survive through becoming my own advocate during my cancer journey. Conversely, I believe that all of the stress and pressure during the years of training would start to take a toll on my health. I hope that the information in this book can help you in whatever journey you might endure in your lifetime. I know that I am repeating myself. Nonetheless, please remember one thing; no matter how severe it gets, someone out there has it much worse than you and I. I focused on this thought many times during my pilgrimage, and the thought helped me handle difficult situations during my fight.

One of the first signs that my health was declining was my platelets dropping below 75,000. Normal platelet counts are 150,000 to 450,000. This was originally detected back in 2008 during kidney stone surgery and was not associated with any cancers. The doctors did not realize that this was a sign because I was otherwise perfectly healthy. This would serve to be another wake-up call, moreover, would lead to other diagnoses.

After five years with J&J, I moved on to Covidien Specialty Pharmaceuticals. My manager Paul moved on to this company after J&J laid him off after 20 plus years. That was one fastidious characteristic about J&J; my division always had layoffs every December. You could be the top rep in the country, and J&J would still displace your job. That is how I was transferred to Knoxville, Tennessee, which was a great city in which to live and work.

Frequent moving is one of the risks that everyone in the medical sales industry takes on for the prestige of the job. I moved three times in five years with J&J, which I feel was a contributing stress on my family. I also feel that the multiple moves and layoffs may of had some effects on my health.

Covidien would train me in every aspect of the pain industry, and we launched two new medications in the pain arena. One of the medications was Exalgo, which was a hydromorphone hydrochloride narcotic for moderate to severe chronic pain. The other medication was Pennsaid which was a topical NSAID (nonsteroidal anti-inflammatory drug) with DMSO or *dimethyl sulfoxide*. We were the first salesforce to launch two medications at the same exact time with the same sales team.

The training and knowledge that I received from Covidien prepared me for my pain management during my almost two year venture. I ended up doing well launching the two medications at Covidien, and I finished third in the nation out of 250 sales reps in 2010 and 25th in the nation in 2011. The two trips I received for President's Cup awards were to Costa Rica and Hawaii. I continued to do well during 2011 even as I was doing radiation and having my multiple surgeries for my cancers.

As 2012 rolled around, I was also doing particularly well. I ended up tenth in the nation out of 245 plus representatives. This was during my AML and MDS battle. Covidien had to let me go in April of 2012 because my short term disability had expired. I will catch everybody up on how to handle financial aspects of having such a devastating disease in upcoming chapters. Remember, that none of this matters when you do not have your health.

Here is a great picture of my friends and partners at Johnson & Johnson enjoying our awards trip in Cabo San Lucas, Mexico. We had an absolute blast. From left to right in the photo is: Lauren, Paul, Jamie, Hal, Asheley, Myself, and George. I sure do miss the great times we had together. Thank you so much for the memories.

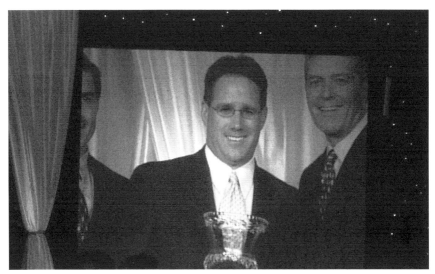

Picture of me receiving my First President's Cup Award at J&J in Cabo San Lucas, Mexico. This was one of the most memorable trips I have ever taken.

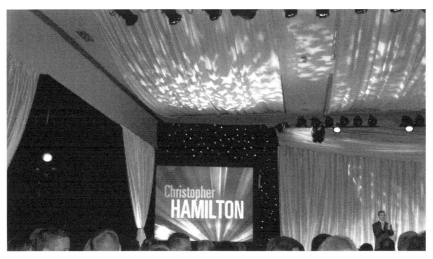

Picture of my name in lights. What a great celebration. Thank you J&J!

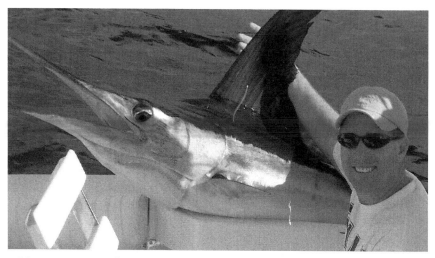

Here is a picture of a striped marlin that I caught off of the coast of Cabo San Lucas. We tagged the Marlin and set him free within minutes. He weighed in at almost 200 pounds and put on a good fight. Little did I know that I would be fighting for my life six years later.

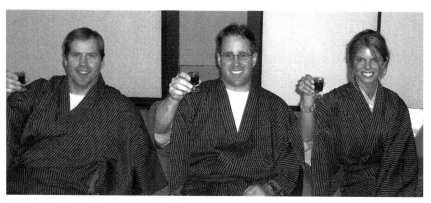

Left to right in the picture: Paul (J&J District Manager), me in the middle and Lauren, J&J Work partner and friend. This is a picture of us enjoying our Japan trip in Kyoto.

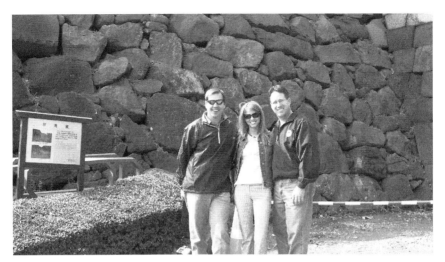

Paul, Lauren and me in front of the Tokyo Imperial Palace in Tokyo, Japan.

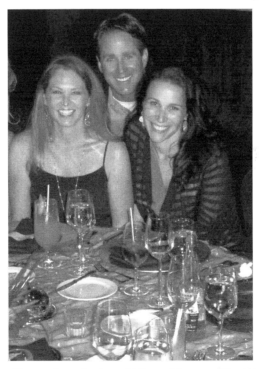

Picture of Laura (Spouse), me in the middle and Lauren (Covidien friend) at my first President's Cup at Covidien. This trip and celebration was in Costa Rica.

CHAPTER 3

BACK TO HOW MY JOURNEY BEGAN

"All journeys have secret destinations of which the traveler is unaware."
Great quotation by Martin Buber.

I soon learned what this quotation meant throughout my two year expedition.

I was sitting in the dentist chair in Southern Pines, North Carolina. Dr. Barry was examining me after my cleaning and mentioned that there was a lesion on my tonsil. Dr. Barry also mentioned that I should definitely get it checked out. I put off my appointment to see my Ear, Nose, and Throat doctor (ENT) for about two weeks until I finally had a second opinion from a friend. Harry, a Physician's Assistant in Raeford, North Carolina, looked at my lesion and told me that I should not put it off any longer.

I then made an appointment with Dr. Pantelakos, an ENT doctor in Fayetteville, North Carolina. The appointment was uneventful, and he said that the lesion looked normal on the surface. Nevertheless, he thought that we should still obtain a biopsy of the lesion. Dr. Pantelakos received the results and said that it came back showing dysplasia or pre-cancer. He said that some people wait but suggested I get a tonsillectomy. I asked him what his next open date for surgery was, and he said April 26, 2011, to which I replied sign me up.

The surgery went well except for the 14 days of extreme pain during the healing process. The process of a tonsillectomy for a child is not that painful. However, for an adult, it is an entirely different story. The pain felt like someone poured acid down my throat 24 hours a day. The tonsils were then analyzed for cancer. The left tonsil came back with squamous cell carcinoma and the margins on paper seemed fine. Dr. Pantelakos suggested I consult my radiologist oncologist in Pinehurst next. Dr. Patel in Pinehurst, informed me that squamous cell carcinoma was very aggressive, and that I should get radiation treatments for my head and neck area.

Something told me that I should get a PET (Positron Emission Tomography) scan next. I wanted to make sure that there was nothing else lurking inside me before I set out to get head and neck radiation. Look, this is an expensive test. However a PET or full body scan will reveal any other cancers that may exist. Please make your doctor discuss this option and what this test can do. I received my results from my PET, and there were two areas of concern. Both areas were in my left thyroid. I next scheduled a needle biopsy for my thyroid in May of 2011, and the biopsy came back as positive for papillary carcinoma of the left thyroid. I then called Dr. Pantelakos and scheduled a surgery to remove my entire thyroid which was my choice. Dr. Pantelakos agreed.

Being that I was a medical rep, I understood that if a patient had cancer on one side of the thyroid, that there would be a high chance of that patient getting cancer on the other side. Why leave tissue to which the cancer can spread when all the he or she needs to do is take a thyroid replacement pill every day for the rest of their life. After the surgery, the biopsy reports came back, and the biopsy confirmed my thought that there was follicular papillary carcinoma on both sides of the thyroid. My intuition was accurate, and I saved myself a second surgery. Always go with your gut, because in the end, your gut is most often right.

My next step was to get an ablation of the thyroid with nuclear medicine. This is common to kill any thyroid cancer cells that may be left over in the body. Then they starved my body of iodine. This seems like an easy task; however, iodine or iodized salt is in almost everything that we consume. They also starved my body of thyroid hormone for one month. This caused hypothyroidism and made me more sluggish than ten chemotherapies at once.

I then received my 103 millicuries of nuclear medicine at Cape Fear Valley Medical Center in Fayetteville, North Carolina. Once I received my dose in pill form, I had to find a location that I could segregate myself from my family. I had to stay in a rental house in Pinehurst for five days. The reason for this was so that my family would not get exposed to radiation. It was live in a separate house, or have my children wear lead lined underwear.

I remember the pain associated with the nuclear medicine leaving my body. The problem was that I was as constipated as Interstate 405 in Southern California, and the nuclear medicine had no way of escaping my body. The main route that nuclear medicine leaves your body is through your feces. I remember sitting on the toilet for three hours one night praying that this terrible nuclear chemical would leave my body. The pain was so excruciating, and it felt like my insides were going to erupt. I thought about dialing 911. But, remember we live in a country where pizza arrives quicker than our emergency services.

Finally, since the nuclear medicine could not leave my body the traditional way, it started leaving my body through sweats and cramps. I then felt the radioactivity leaving through my hands, and they had a sticky substance on them for the next few days. It was like something out of a science fiction movie. After the three hours of pain and suffering; the constipation gave way. Thank God I was then able to pass on most of the radioactivity, and I started feeling better.

I then felt it was to a good time to get a second and third opinion for my head and neck radiation. I scheduled a trip with my family to travel up to Connecticut. This worked out great because I could go to Yale New Haven Cancer Hospital, and travel to New York to enjoy a trip with my family. I saw the Department Head, Dr. Son, an ENT with a primary focus on head and neck cancers. After I discussed all of my notes with Dr. Son, he examined me thoroughly. I remember Dr. Son saying, "If this were me, I would do six and half weeks of radiation in the left tonsil area, and make sure you have them treat no more than 54 GY." Dr. Son was definitely worth the trip and one of the most astute doctors I had the pleasure of meeting during my tour.

I also figured that I would get a third opinion before I had Moore Regional Radiation Oncologist Dr. Patel treat me. So I made an appointment to see a leader in head and neck surgery for my last opinion. My gut was telling me not to do the radiation. Nonetheless, everyone that I had an appointment with told me the same thing; squamous cell carcinoma is aggressive and not to be fooled with at all. My third opinion came from Dr. Weissler at the University of North Carolina (UNC) Head and Neck Cancer Department.

Dr. Weissler also suggested six and half weeks of head and neck radiation. Three opinions were enough for me; I needed to bite the bullet and go through the radiation. I then thought to myself, once I complete my six and half weeks of intensive head and neck radiation, I would be finished with my cancer treatments. This is when the plot really thickens, and my journey would start to take shape.

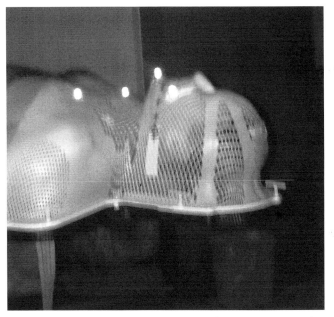

This is a picture of one radiation treatment out of my 32 received. The weirdest feeling about the treatments was my head being pinned down and not being able to move for the 20 minutes. The burns were also intense and painful towards the end. They custom fit the harness to secure your head and neck perfectly. If you are at all claustrophobic, talk to your radiation oncologist to get a medication to help with relaxing you. I talked with a few patients in the waiting room every morning that had to sedate themselves to deal with being restrained during every treatment.

CHAPTER 4

11/11/11 AND HOW MY LIFE TOOK A TURN

"Nothing in fine print is ever good news" Great quotation From Andy Rooney.

I asked myself many of times, "is this bad news disguised as good news?" After reading my book, you will understand what I mean.

Five and half weeks into my six and half week head and neck radiation treatments, and I started feeling ill. Dr. Patel always did blood work every week to make sure that everything was going as planned. During the last five days of my treatments, my white blood cell count and platelets took a dive and I starting feeling ill.

Dr. Patel was concerned, and wanted me to get a second opinion from another oncologist in Fayetteville. The oncologist I saw told me that I should complete my radiation and hope that my numbers recover. Dr. Patel was hesitant on completing my treatments. However, she commented that if I did not complete a course of radiation, there was a good chance that the treatment would not be effective. I had come too far; I need to complete my treatments.

We continued my treatments, and my blood count numbers continued to decrease. After completing all of my radiation treatments, a skin infection appeared on my leg. The skin infection was so critical that they hospitalized me to treat me with Vancomycin, one of the most potent and best antibiotics available. Vancomycin treated the MRSA *Methicillin-resistant Staphylococcus Aureus* on my leg. Dr. Moore, my Oncologist in Pinehurst, was my attending oncologist during my stay. He tried to treat my low blood numbers with Neupogen shots, which boosts white blood cells (WBC). My numbers only recovered enough to get me a ticket out of the hospital.

After being discharged from the hospital, I visited my good friend Dan Matthews, PA-C. Dan is my family's physician. Dan checked my blood to see if my numbers returned to normal. Dan received the numbers back the next day, and he informed me that things had worsened. Dan said that he was going to call Dr. Moore and request that a bone marrow biopsy be completed on me in the next couple of days.

Dr. Moore scheduled a bone marrow biopsy right away, and he completed it the following week in early November 2011. The bone marrow biopsy is accomplished by drilling into your back area, above your buttocks. First the hematologist administers some sedation with pain medication to numb the bone. Then they drill into the bone with a hollow needle. Once the needle is in the bone, they then suction out a marrow and a blood sample.

Dr. Moore received my results on 11/11/11, and called me with what I knew was truly bad news or was it bad news? This always depends on how one views the news. He said, "Chris your results came back, and show 27% blasts and you are positive for AML [Acute Myelogenous Leukemia]."

Dr. Moore also told me that the AML was one of the most aggressive forms of leukemia that I could have, AML M2. AML is a form of blood and marrow cancer that can take your life in the matter of two months without treatment. Dr. Moore said, "you can select Duke or UNC Cancer Hospital; whichever you choose, you will have to be there by this evening to start treatments." I was devastated. I thought for a moment that I had completed all of my fighting. It had been 8 months since discovering my tonsil cancer and I had since gone through multiple tests and torturous treatments. But, Dr. Moore had just told me that my battle had just begun.

I imagine that discovering I had AML must feel like a person losing his or her home to foreclosure or perhaps discovering that he or she has months to live and to see his or her kids. Many thoughts were running through my head. I felt alone, violated, and cursed. I had feelings of mediocrity. And, for the first time, I did not know enough about a disease state to help myself. I felt like I had two left feet, and suddenly I forgot how to dance. I felt like I was drowning in a lake of fear. This was my life we were talking about here.

It was 4:00pm. My spouse Laura and son Brennan had already departed for a soccer tournament in Richmond, Virginia. I called Laura and explained my diagnosis, and that I needed to be at UNC within the next few hours. She felt like collapsing in the lobby of the hotel and could not believe the news. I then packed a suitcase because I knew that the first chemotherapy involved was going to be tough. I also knew that the first of many treatments lasted 30 plus days in the hospital.

I called Aaron, a friend that I knew was in town for a haircut. Aaron was my climbing buddy, and a pain doctor that I called on in Fayetteville. I explained my diagnosis and told him that I had three hours to get to UNC Cancer Hospital. Aaron said, "No problem Chris, I will be there in 15 minutes, get your bags packed." Aaron arrived to pick me up, and he had tears in his eyes. Aaron understood the severity of the diagnosis, and he knew that I probably would have another year of treatments. Aaron also knew the recovery to beat this awful disease would be several months. He tried kidding around with me by saying, "this is a lousy way to get out of rock climbing every weekend." Not funny Aaron.

Aaron drove Riley and me to UNC Cancer Center in Chapel Hill, North Carolina. I checked in at the front desk and I was in the state of shock. They had a room ready for me within minutes. Family started flying in that night, one after another. The nurses and doctors were swarming my room making me seriously nervous.

I will never forget the first night on 11/11/11. The time was about 11:30pm, and I guess the stress and the shock hit me like a ton of bricks squarely in the chest. My chest started getting tight. My throat started closing in on me. I had a sharp pain on the left side of my ribcage. It felt like someone was driving a knife into the side of my chest. I called the nurse and explained that my chest was hurting, and before I could blink my eyes, there was a total of 16 medical staff in my room.

The nurse hit the code button, and the entire floor seemed to have appeared in my room. You know when you are in the hospital and you hear, "Code red, all available staff to room . . . ."? Well, when you hear that this is what is occurring. More staff than is easily counted is descending upon one person who may or may not be conscious. I was conscious, and all I was thinking was that everybody was staring at me in my boxers. I was too busy worrying about having a Sharon Stone moment during all of this excitement and panic. Could you imagine my junk falling out in front of ten plus female nurses?

This caused me to be non-responsive to many of their questions. They gave me two milligrams of Ativan intravenously to relax me, and they were throwing 1,000 questions at me. They rushed equipment into every bit of space left in the room. They asked that all of family wait in the hall and then started hooking me up to EKG machines, cardiac echo machines, mobile x-ray machines, etc.

I tried to explain to them that this was stress induced and that I had never had a heart attack in my life. One of the doctors looked at me and said, "Well guess what, you experienced a mild heart attack or event." Eventually things would calm down around 3:00am. The nurse came in and asked me to get some rest because tomorrow would be an entire day of tests for your heart. She said, "We cannot give you your induction chemotherapy until we clear your heart." Wow, what a first night at UNC. I explained to the nurses that I enjoy making an entrance, so that everybody knows that I am in the house. They all laughed and said we like you Chris.

I could not believe that I was diagnosed, and that my results came back on 11/11/11. I cannot tell you how many times that 11/11 came up in my life; maybe as many as 25 times during memorable events.

Why has 111 or 1111 come up so much in my life? What did all this mean? Laura and I were married on the 111th day of the year, April 20, 1992. We moved our wedding date up six months because of Laura's Grandfather being diagnosed with cancer. I met Laura on January 11, 1991 (01/11/91).

There have been many other examples throughout my life. When looking back on all of these coincidences or events, I finally came to the conclusion that many of these 1111 events were warning signs. I also concluded that I was on the wrong track in life. I felt strongly that I needed to refocus my energy and work on my stress levels. Well, certainly mark 1111 events as being one my *CHE-MOments* in my journey.

Before moving on, I feel this is a great time to discuss cancer in more detail for those that have not experienced the diagnosis. I also want to discuss it more for the caregivers and family, because cancer can mean so many different things to the person fighting. If you are the fighter; furthermore, this might help you feel that your emotions are the same as many other people. The importance of life and priorities completely changes. Many people experience different stages or emotional changes. When talking to many of my fellow fighters, they emphasized the following as being important to them; quality of life, closing loose ends, visiting people that they have not seen in a while, getting closer to God, confronting demons/fears, and some were just plain mad and upset at the world. Some blamed God and some blamed family for their diagnoses.

Please contemplate all of the above before judging anyone that is in the middle of his or her fight. I looked at my diagnosis as a gift or a chance to do many of the items listed above. Please do not waste any energy on blaming anyone for your diagnosis. Please focus on what is important to you. Because your time on this earth is in question. As you continue to read my book, everything will start to make sense, and you will see that my priorities changed a few times during my pilgrimage. I hope that helps everyone understand a little more about cancer and how the importance changes from person to person. Please be as understanding as you can with everybody involved, because cancer can tear families apart or cancer can pull families closer together.

My journey starts to take shape in the next chapter, so buckle up. I also discuss more detail around attitude towards cancer. Enjoy this quotation.

"Life is too short to start your day with broken pieces of yesterday, it will definitely destroy your wonderful today, and ruin your great tomorrow." Unknown Author

CHAPTER 5

MO-HAWK AND READY TO TAKE ON THE FIGHT/JOURNEY

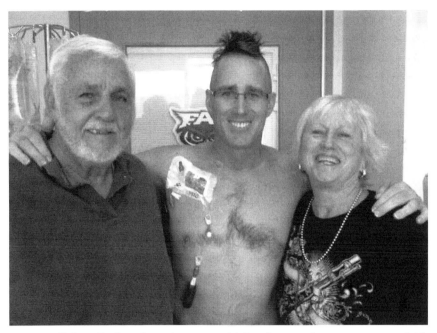

Picture of Mom, Dad, and me during my 24-7 induction chemo treatment which is the first of many chemo treatments. Sporting the MO-Hawk, and ready to start my next leg of my trek. I figured my hair was falling out anyway, so why not have a little fun. Riley and Brennan loved it.

"Cancer is a word, not a sentence!" John Diamond. Remember that you can look at cancer as a blessing or you can look at cancer as a burden/sentence. This is a great time to start looking into your life, reflect, and keep your chin up. There are only two paths a cancer patient can take. Why not make it the path of positive thoughts, prayer, meditation, and miracles? Why not tell yourself that you are not going to let cancer bring you down? Why not exercise each day during your venture? Exercise, prayer, meditation, and good attitude sure did help me.

During my journey many people asked me how chemotherapy felt. I can best describe leukemia chemotherapy as the following: it leaves you bald, dried-out, pimpled, it makes you nauseated, makes you feel tired, makes you lose weight, it makes your mouth and throat shed, it gives you sores in your mouth that become excruciating, it weakens your lungs, and makes concentrating difficult, and most of all it kills your immune system. I lost 40 pounds during my six plus months of chemotherapy. The chemotherapy you receive before stem cell transplant is the most brutal chemotherapy available. Many people also asked me questions on cancer and how it affect us.

My friend Valeria gave me a great insight to shed light on cancer, and how we can let cancer affect us. She said, "There are three options; you can surrender and let cancer destroy not only your physical body but your spirit also. You can let cancer destroy the spirit but not the body. Or, you can make cancer your ally and key to positive beginnings." Valeria is a great friend and smart. She and I discussed cancer at length many of times. You ever listen to *Paul Simon's song The Boxer*. The lyrics that jump out at me every time I hear it is:

"In the clearing stands a boxer
And a fighter by his trade
And he carries the remainders
Of every glove that laid him down
And cut him till he cried out
In his anger and his shame
"I am leaving, I am leaving"
But the fighter still remains"

This is what I want you to carry with you—no matter what cancer throws at you, please be the fighter that remains. I cannot tell you how many people on the cancer floor would just close the shades, get into the fetal position, and admit defeat. You have to ask yourself what do I have to live for? I say we have plenty. You could live for your kids, your family, your mom, and your dad. You could live for wanting to see your college football team play one more time. Maybe you could live for ocean fishing, horseback riding, climbing, hiking, fly fishing, painting, photography, surfing, hockey, soccer; whatever your passion may be. If you are in the middle of your venture right now, I want you to start visualizing what you are going to do when you are healthy. I focused on fly fishing with my boy's Riley and Brennan. Fly fishing relaxes me, and I found that it is a great way for me to decrease my stress levels.

I also visualized how I was going to help people, or reach as many of people as I could with my survival tips. Being in the hospital is tough work, because you can never let your guard down. When you are receiving chemo and your numbers are dropping it is tough to do everything required of you.

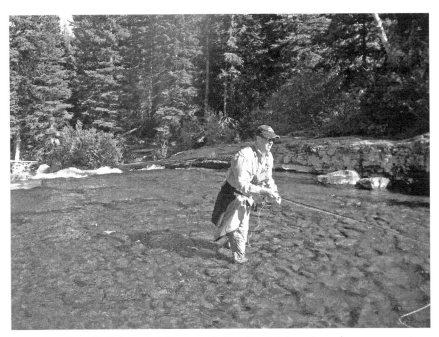

Picture of me fly fishing in Montana. I visualized this daily to focus on positive energy of curing my AML and MDS.

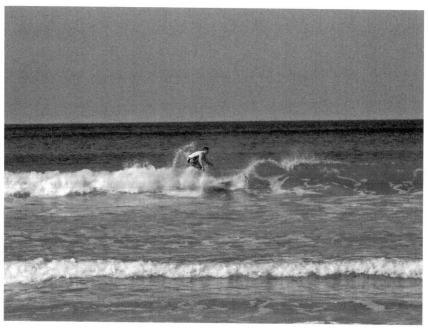

Here is a picture of me surfing in Costa Rica during my 2011 President's Cup win with Covidien. I also visualized surfing to pass my time during my hospital stays. I also played my i-Pod each day to relax, and that always put me in a positive state of mind.

You must keep track of the medications that you take. I suggest you keep a list of medications and the strengths listed. If you are fighting AML or any other Leukemia/cancer, you could be on as many as 20 medications, especially if you are in the middle of transplant. The one thing I want you to remember is that nurses and doctors are human, and they can make mistakes. I caught two medication mistakes during my many hospital stays. Too much thyroid medication one morning and your thyroid levels could be out of sorts for up to a week. Too many medications excreted through the kidneys, and your creatine clearance could be elevated for the week. Too many medications excreted through the liver, and your enzymes can be elevated. Small mistakes can put your cancer treatments on hold for days and sometimes weeks.

It is always best to write down questions for the attending doctor each day, especially if you are in a teaching hospital. If you are in a teaching hospital; I suggest limiting the number of people in your room during your stay. I have had as many as 10 doctors and nurses in my room at once, and when you are receiving chemotherapy or recovering from chemo, your immune system is completely exposed. You have to be your own advocate, and I will mention this several times throughout the book in hopes that it limits the mistakes made during your comeback.

Do not be afraid to ask the nurses questions before they do procedures on you. If fighting AML or other blood cancers, nurses will change out your port needles every seven days. The UNC Cancer Hospital has 48 beds on 4th floor Oncology (4-Onc). As you could imagine, this could expose you to a variety of nurses. Occasionally you will get a nurse that is rather fresh out of school. The reason I bring this up is that this is where mistakes can happen. Remember that everyone is human. Do not be afraid to request their most senior nurse to do major procedures on you.

The first major mistake with my first induction chemo treatments was a needle change out or dressing change for my dual power port. This was the first week after I had been admitted, and I was never told what to do or to be my own advocate. I had a nurse that was a few months out of training. She claimed that she was the best at needle changes for power ports. I trusted her, and I have always been respectful of all people taking care of me. This nurse tried to place the first needle in my port, and she missed the port all together puncturing my muscle layer in my chest. The pain was intense! These ports tend to move around a bit. Furthermore, it is important for them to hold the port still. She said, "I am sorry let me try again." It took the nurse four more tries to hit the port, and she finally placed the first of the two needles. I also noticed that she became nervous, and she touched the side of the bed once with her gloves. "Oh crap!" I knew the importance of staying sterile during needle placement, and I thought to myself this could be an issue. In her defense, my chest area was already swollen because of the fresh port placement a few days earlier. She asked for the nurse manager to come in, and she was able to place the second needle on the first try. Please be sure to learn from my mistakes, and request someone else after they miss with your port needles. There is no reason to endure more pain above what you are already going through with your cancers.

Guess what happened from me being too quiet and letting the nurse poke me five times? I received a port infection within 24 hours. This port infection caused me to extend my hospital stay by another seven days, and I needed to receive Vancomycin antibiotic through my port. In turn, my creatine clearance sky rocketed from the multiple drugs being excreted through my kidneys. Now my treatments were put off another week because of one mistake.

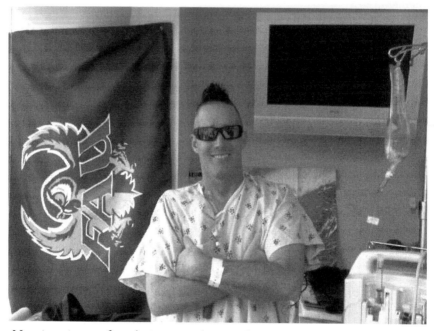

Here is a picture of me during my induction chemo sporting my new MO-hawk and Brennan's sun glasses. My family also decorated my room for my first five week stay at UNC Cancer Center. As you can see, I was also sporting my FAU flag. Florida Atlantic University is my Alma Mater, and I am proud of my school. I was walking up to two miles a day around 4-Onc with my new walking buddy Ricky. Ricky was also diagnosed with AML a couple of months before me.

From that day forward I was my own advocate, and I stayed on top of everything that went on with my treatments.

Another great piece of advice is to get as much exercise that you can get, and stay in the best possible shape. There will be days that you do not ever want to get out of bed and days that it takes everything you have to get up and exercise. During my induction chemotherapy, which lasted 40 days because of the infection, I made it a point to walk at least one and a half to two miles per day. Most cancer floors should have a walking area. UNC had an area in which you could walk in the hallways during certain hours. Exercise not only helped me keep my spirits up, it also helped me comeback quicker from each of the many chemotherapies.

One of my bone marrow coordinators, Martha, had one the best sayings that stuck with me throughout my journey. She would ask, "Would you rather be a babbling brook or a still pond?" Then Martha would follow by saying, "What happens in still ponds? Still ponds are always green and full of bacteria and babbling brooks are always clear, moving, and healthy." That made enough of an impression with me that I always exercised, even through my transplant.

Your doctor, nurse, physical therapist, and recreational therapist can work together to come up with an exercise plan that is perfect for you. Besides walking each day, the following exercises are also important and worth asking about; straight leg raise, hip extension, quadricep extension, hip abduction, toe raises, and hamstring flexes. A great DVD to purchase is *Lee Holden's, Qi Gong for Low Back Pain.* The reason I bring this DVD up is that it encompasses the exercises listed above and meditation. It is also important to remember your lungs during and after your chemotherapies and transplant too. The best way to strengthen your lungs is to ask for an incentive spirometer to use throughout your stay, and use it religiously. Another great website for these exercises is *http://www.mayoclinic.com/health/stretching*.

Here is another great tip if you have been diagnosed with AML. Please file for Social Security Disability (SSD) immediately. It takes at least three months to get your benefits. One silver lining about a devastating diagnosis like AML is that SSD will approve your benefits when they receive your doctor's notes and files. I received an approval for my benefits in two weeks. However, it was four months before I received actual money. Another suggestion is to try and get your current employer to extend any short-term disability benefits to you and avoid losing your job at all costs.

I will touch upon many aspects of financial consequences throughout the book because cancer diagnoses can be financially draining.

Total bills for my transplant, scans, bone marrow biopsies, hospital stays, surgeries, port placements, port removals, infections, medications, gas, and parking at hospitals was well over $2,000,000. Total co-pays, deductibles, and expenses not covered through medical insurance, COBRA, and SSD came to about $30,000 out of pocket over a two year period. Just to clarify, I had private insurance. If you have Medicaid or Medicare your costs will be much lower.

Do not freak out because there are secrets to keeping those out-of-pocket expenses affordable. While I remember, a great nonprofit organization to utilize is The Bone Marrow Foundation in New York. They can set up a One-to-One fund, so that your friends and loved ones can send tax deductible donations to the fund for you. You can pay for medications, medical bills, co-pays, parking, etc. The Foundation only receives a small hold back to operate their nonprofit. The holdback or percentage they kept was only 5%.

One other tip is to make sure that you request a social worker be assigned to you during your hospital stays at the cancer hospital at which you get your treatments, etc. The social worker will help you navigate through all the financial questions you may have and will have a list of great organizations out there with money for cancer patients.

The Leukemia and Lymphoma Society usually has $100 available for each year that you are fighting blood or bone cancers. A hundred dollars may not seem like much. Nevertheless, every little bit helps. If not managed properly, this disease can financially devastate a family. Be the Match also has money available for stem cell transplant patients after you receive your transplant, and it usually is around $500 to $1,500.

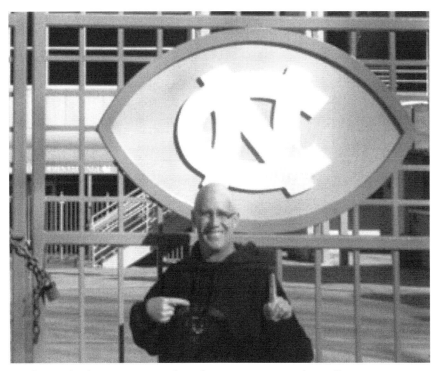

Getting back to exercising; please be sure to get outside as often as you can. Unfortunately, cancer hospitals only allow you to travel outside when your numbers are up: ANC, WBC, platelets, etc. When you are able and your numbers are good, get up and get out. Getting outside will do so much for you and your attitude. That fresh air and humidity will do you some good, trust me.

Here is a picture of me in front of Kenan Memorial Stadium (home of UNC Football). I am pointing to my sweatshirt which shows FAU, making sure everyone knows that I am still a FAU fan through thick and thin. I often went on long walks from UNC Hospital to Franklin Street with my wife Laura. This was a three mile round trip walk, and the walk did so much for me emotionally and physically.

I also made it a point to participate in the activities that the cancer floor would have set up each day. I did arts and crafts, participated in support groups, and visited with as many people as I could; depending on my numbers. I also asked that someone from the local Catholic church bring me communion every Sunday or a few times a week. Try to live as normal of a life as you can because the comeback will be that much easier. If you do not get out and exercise each day, at least walk. Otherwise, you stand the chance of atrophy. Depending on your age, atrophy can hit quickly. In the case of a person in his or her mid 40s, atrophy can take over in the matter of one week. I know I said this before, but make sure your blinds stay open and you stay active. A beautiful sunrise could make your day. Remember we are like lizards. We thrive on many benefits that the sun provides.

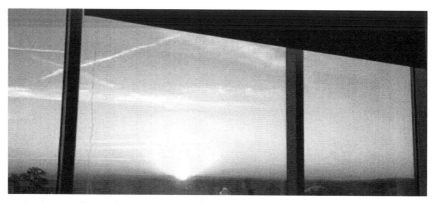

A picture of one of many sunrises that I experienced from my room at UNC Cancer Hospital. If I had my blinds closed, I would have never been exposed to such a gift and beauty from God. Through exercise, meditation, prayer, and positive attitude you too have a better chance of beating your cancer. Remember, I had less than a 25% chance and crushed the odds.

I will discuss meditation later in the book because it will be important to your journey and beating the odds.

CHAPTER 6

DO NOT SWEAT THE SMALL STUFF—DARK DAYS AND BAD NEWS

"The woods are lovely, dark, and deep. But I have promises to keep, and miles to go before I sleep."—Robert Frost

Robert Frost was brilliant, and this quotation from one of his poems has never left me since high school. Have you heard the expression that your job or task is meant to be thought of as a marathon and not as a sprint? That is what I want you to think about during your journey. Look, this may not be a journey that you would choose; no one would choose this. Your lack of choice is now irrelevant. Like it or not, your journey has begun. The sooner you embrace the journey, the easier it will become to endure the trek. We are meant to go through this pilgrimage, so saddle up and make the best of it.

When you come out on the other side of your trek, or out of the woods, you will have a gift that few will have the chance to experience in their lifetimes. This gift I speak of is a constant reminder of thanks and gratitude. I cannot explain this to you because it is beyond words. Rather, here is my quotation that may shed light on it:

"We must acknowledge what God has given us, and be forever grateful for it today, tomorrow, and every day forward."
—Chris J. Hamilton

I thank God every day for the beauty in this world; seeing my kids grow-up, being able to share my experience with you, being able to help people realize that the petty stuff they complain about does not matter, etc. I stay in contact with another AML survivor Jonathan, three years post-transplant, and I asked him if this feeling ever goes away. Jonathan says that it only gets stronger and stronger as time grows.

Jonathan was my mentor during the transplant process, and I was blessed to have such an outlet. You too can get a mentor through The Bone Marrow Foundation in New York.

I heard another person explain that you have to think of your journey as taking two steps forward, and then taking one step back. The explanation for this, is that some people's bodies cannot take the many medications and or chemo that are required to beat these diseases. Further, if you are fighting AML or cancer, uncomfortable news is part of the routine.

The one step back might be that you have something go wrong with your spleen or another organ. Do not worry, everyone will experience something along the way, and the important thing is to remember to keep your chin-up. If your donor was a perfect match, the side effects and graft versus host (GVH) usually stay at a minimum. Remember that there is always someone out there going through more than you are dealing with; it is the way you deal with it that counts! In addition, I believe that God watches us to see how we handle adversity/pain and then rewards us if we are worthy.

When I was diagnosed with my AML, it was classified as M2. M2 is one of the toughest blood cancers to treat, especially if your cytogenetics are bad or if you also have Myelodysplastic Syndrome (MDS). AML affects 13,000 people annually in the United States. Nine-thousand of them die.

After my first chemotherapy induction treatment, I was also diagnosed with MDS. MDS produces abnormal cells in your blood and marrow. The doctor explained my case as being one of the toughest to treat on the floor of 48 beds in 4-Onc. Wow, the worst out of 48 patients—that cannot be good. Remember, keep your chin up.

One of the great aspects of UNC is that they collaborate with M.D. Anderson on the latest and greatest in treatments available for blood cancer. The doctor also explained that my case would take a little longer to cure or to hit remission. She further explained that the only way my cure could come is if I were to undergo a stem cell transplant once I reach remission. Without a stem cell transplant, my life expectancy would have been two months.

My next dark day or piece of bad news would come as more chemo failures. If you are fighting any form of blood cancer, you too may fail many chemotherapies. Hang in there, this is your road to travel. Not only did I fail my induction chemo, I failed the next few chemotherapies they tried on me. My first induction chemo ended in December, and my first hospital stay lasted over 40 days.

Remember that saying, Two steps forward and one step back. Even though I was failing the chemotherapies, I was still fighting the disease and making progress or taking steps forward. My blast levels or cancerous cells were heading down; however, they would never drop below 16%. This meant that my blood and marrow contained 16% cancer cells in my body.

After my first chemo failure, UNC scheduled another round in January 2012, which would be another two week hospital stay. I was lucky enough to have a great cancer hospital in Pinehurst and was able to receive some of my follow-up treatments and transfusions. If I did not have First Health Out Patient Cancer Center in Pinehurst, I would have been forced to stay at UNC for three to four weeks at a time.

My bone marrow biopsy results came in after my second round of chemotherapy and my blast levels did not budge, still at 16%. I questioned my doctors at UNC because I was concerned. Dr. Richards, trained at M.D. Anderson, said that she had a salvage chemo regimen that M.D. Anderson was experimenting with and that the regimen seemed to be working on many tough to treat cases.

My salvage chemo would be scheduled in February 2012, and it would definitely put me to the test. This was a chemo treatment which used steroids, Neupogen shots, and two powerful chemotherapies. I again stayed in the hospital for two weeks and then went home for my transfusions after the treatments. I had another bone marrow biopsy completed to see how the salvage chemotherapy worked. Another failure; my blasts came in above 11%. What is going on? Why do I keep failing all of these chemotherapies? Now I was starting to get concerned. Nevertheless, I continued to keep my chin up. How much more can my liver, lungs, and spleen take from these terrible chemicals and poison?

Soon after I failed several rounds of chemotherapy and one round of intensive salvage chemo, it was time for a family vacation. I had come to the point during my treatments in which I said to myself that this is not how I want my boys to remember me. I scheduled a vacation against my doctor's wishes; a wonderful vacation down in Marco Island. I wanted this to be a great fun filled vacation and a break from the, so far, one year venture from my cancers. I wanted my wife Laura and my boys Riley and Brennan to enjoy and always remember my journey to have some breaks along the way. Life is short. Please enjoy what you can each and every day.

I booked a suite in the Marco Island Marriott overlooking the ocean. I told the kids that we were going to blow it out and do whatever they wished. This was going to be a great trip, and I could not wait to get away from all of the hospitals and needles. You have to recharge your battery during your fight, or you will not have enough in the tank to continue.

What patients have to remember is that doctors live in a bubble. Moreover, they only practice out of a book and have a difficult time putting themselves in your shoes. They sometimes forget about the human aspect of treating a patient. My doctors at UNC were not comfortable with me going on vacation. Nonetheless, I knew a vacation was what my family needed. Dr. Moore, however, was not one of those doctors that lived in the bubble. He understood me and agreed that I should enjoy some time and recharge the battery.

So we did, and the trip was absolutely incredible. My boys and I rode jet skis, and ate the best grouper sandwiches. We also drank nonalcoholic piña coladas next to the pool and near the ocean. I gave them endless money to play in the video game area. We played a hundred games of ping pong, and money was no question at this point. We lived life like it was 1999, *Prince song*. We definitely emptied some of the bucket list on this trip, and I wanted no regrets while fighting these diagnoses.

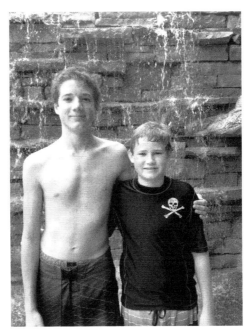

Riley on left and Brennan on right. Enjoying the trip of a lifetime. We had a blast!

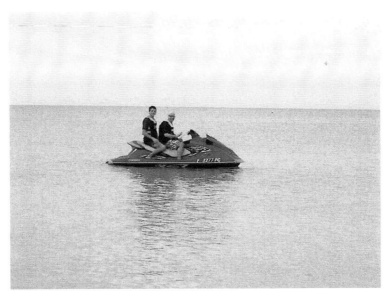

Here is a picture of Riley and me on a jet ski at Marco Island. The ocean was perfect that day, and we had an awesome time. I think we exceeded speeds of 60 MPH, and I showed him a few tricks of my own.

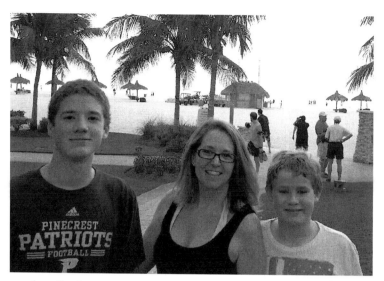

Picture of my family enjoying a sunset at the Marriott in Marco Island. From left to right; Riley, Laura, and Brennan. The weather was perfect the entire vacation, and this trip was exactly what my family needed during the two year journey. The Marriott even played movies on the beach at night.

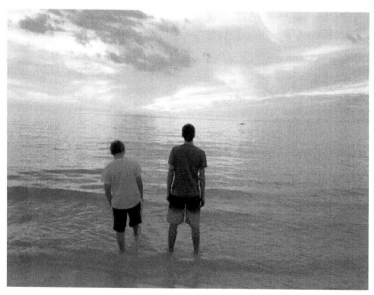

Brennan and Riley enjoying another great sunset. I am so blessed to have spent this memorable time with my family. There is always time for rest during your fight. As you can see that God is ever present in this photo.

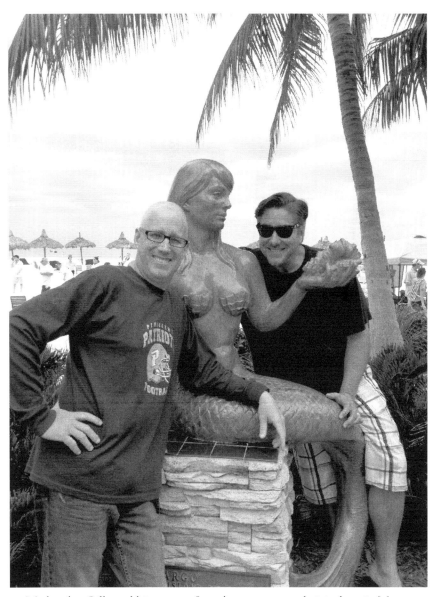

My brother Billy and his partner Joseph came over and visited me in Marco Island. Here is a picture of Billy after we ate a great lunch on the ocean. They brought me a great bouquet of flowers and many gifts to help me through my venture. They assured me that I would be fine and that I would beat this terrible disease. Billy and Joseph told me from the beginning that I would walk away from all of these cancers.

Please be sure to take a break in your treatments, especially if the opportunity presents itself. I want to also repeat myself that you will have bad days and or bad news. However, it is how you deal with that bad news which can affect the outcome. It is important to manage your stress because keeping a positive mind can improve your chances.

"I have heard there are troubles of more than one kind. Some come from ahead, and some come from behind, but I have bought a big bat. I am all ready you see. Now my troubles are going to have troubles with me!" Dr. Seuss

Carry a BIG BAT during your journey and do not let bad news hold you down long, because good news is just around the corner.

CHAPTER 7

WHY ARE THERE NOT ANY PICTURES OF AML SURVIVORS IN THE UNC CANCER LOBBY

During my salvage chemo in February and during other chemotherapies, I often took strolls outside or down to the lobby. UNC also had a labyrinth outside of the cancer hospital, which I spent many hours walking and praying. The UNC Lineberger Cancer Hospital Labyrinth is pictured below.

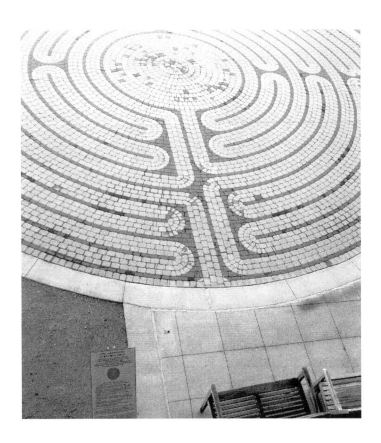

As I had mentioned before, you must get outside when your numbers are adequate to take advantage of the fresh air. If you have the benefit of a labyrinth, please take advantage of it by meditating or praying during your pilgrimage.

While we are on the subject of meditation, I highly recommend that you practice some form of resting your mind. Best time to do meditation is during a quiet part of the day. The best time in a teaching hospital is during shift changes or when the doctors are doing their grand rounds. You can do meditation with music or without music. Make sure to get into a comfortable position, and that may be lying down on your back. Take in deep breaths while sitting still and focus on your breathing. Relax your muscles, your eyes, and your mind. Forget about where you are. You can think about your favorite relaxing hobby or think about the sound of the water crashing on the beach. You can focus on the sound of a stream slowly winding down the mountains.

I know this sounds cliché. But, try to be one with what you are picturing in your mind. Think about being somewhere where it is quiet; no work, no bills, no responsibilities, no fear, and no cancer. Have only positive thoughts of getting well and living life on your terms.

You need to take breaks during each day and rest the mind. If you do not take breaks, the stress will consume you. If you cannot focus on meditation; at least play some music and close your eyes. Relax and try focusing on your breathing. As mentioned before, chemotherapy is destructive to your lungs, and breathing exercises are important.

Just as meditation is important to your well-being, I also want to share with you some of my thoughts around praying for a cure. Not once did I ever pray for a cure. Furthermore, I felt that would be selfish. What I did pray about everyday was for God to give me strength, and for God to give me guidance. After I failed so many chemotherapies, I prayed diligently that God would please give me guidance on what to do next? My doctors were at a loss and did not know what or where to go next. This was another reason why I took that vacation to Marco Island with the family. The time away would give my doctors time to reach out to other cancer institutions and come up with the next step.

During one of my strolls with Laura, I took the time to read all of the survivor stories and pictures in the UNC lobby. This took us about an hour, and it was great to read how everybody fought and won. About three quarters of the way through reading all the success stories, I broke down and cried right there in the lobby. As you will find out, chemotherapies make you an emotional wreck and this one that really hit me hard.

Laura asked what was wrong and held me in her arms. I explained that we read 25 success stories about everyone's cancer journeys, and NOT ONE was about an AML cancer survivor. I asked Laura why. Why are there no damn success stories? Am I fighting a losing battle? Is this disease really that devastating? Laura replied, "UNC may have overlooked this, and maybe they have not had an AML patient to allow them to include their story."

After I collected my thoughts and wiped my tears away; I looked at Laura and told her that my picture was going to be the first AML survivor in the UNC lobby. Damn it, I want my picture in this lobby today so that I can give hope to every AML patient that walks through these doors.

I marched up stairs to tell my bone marrow coordinator, Debbie, the story. I also told her that she needed to get the photographer ready. She laughed and said, "Chris you are rare, and I am sure that we will get that done when you complete you stem cell transplant and kick AML's butt." Unfortunately, UNC removed all the pictures in the lobby and returned the pictures to the survivors in August of 2012.

This is the attitude you need to carry with you during your journey. Remember, that no matter what hits you, you cannot let it keep you down on the ground. You must get up, dust off your hospital gown, and continue to fight. YOU CAN DO THIS! I know you can! **You don't know how strong you are, until being strong is the only choice you have.**" Unknown Author

Instead of my picture in the lobby, I did get a surprise from UNC. My quilt tile that I created during my transplant is now hanging in the Bone Marrow unit lobby. The quilt was for the 20th Anniversary of the Bone Marrow Program at UNC.

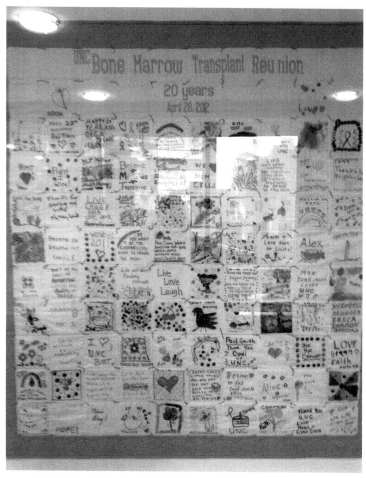

A picture of 20th Anniversary Quilt for the Bone Marrow Transplant Program at UNC Cancer Hospital. The next picture shows a close-up of my tile.

My tile (below) read *Any Goal worth reaching for never comes without hard work, sweat, and tears.*

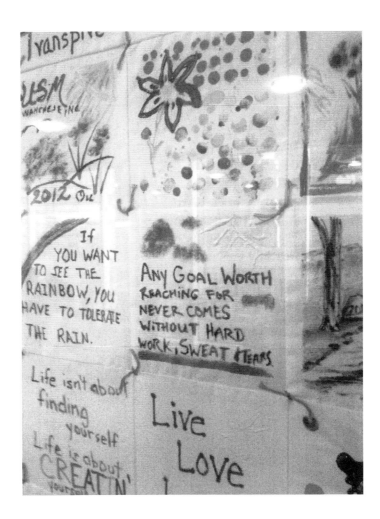

I know that my artistic talent is lacking. Nonetheless, my feelings were accurate on that day. I made this tile three days before my transplant, and my thoughts/hands were not stable because of all the medications and lack of sleep. I never thought that it would be placed in the center of their 20th Anniversary Quilt. What a wonderful surprise to see many months after my transplant. Thank you UNC!

CHAPTER 8

PLAN B, BIG DECISIONS, AND LAST RIGHTS

"When God is going to do something wonderful, He always starts with a hardship; when God is going to do something amazing, He starts with an impossibility."
—Anne Lamott

I would say that having a less than 25% chance could be considered an impossibility by some. But, I was not going to be another AML statistic. Because of all the repeated chemo failures, I needed to formulate a Plan B. The reason I call it Plan B, is that sometimes in your fight you will start to worry about spending healthy/quality time with family. I have mentioned that I have two beautiful Sons, and I this is why I started worrying after failing three chemo regimens. Then after my fourth chemotherapy round, which was my salvage chemo failed, it was time to rethink my plans or develop that Plan B.

My medical insurance nurse also called me a few days before, wanting to give a list of hospice locations. This was because of my consistent chemo failures. That really hit home with me, and made me feel that Plan B was necessary. Both in-network options for hospice were located in Southern Pines.

I then talked to my Oncologist in Pinehurst, Dr. Moore, and explained how I felt. I told him that my last 10 months have been fighting for my life and constantly coming back from chemotherapies. That is the hardest side effect of chemo; having zero energy and having zero immune system. I felt that my life had become nothing but chemotherapy, transfusions, and hospital stays. He talked with my doctors at UNC, and they came up with another plan.

Dr. Moore explained that there is one drug called Decitabine or Dacogen. You can take monthly and live for about 10 to 12 months, and then pass on. He said that this drug is utilized to treat MDS, which I was also fighting. He also said that Decitabine is a more mild chemotherapy drug that many older patients take. The reason for this is that an older patient cannot handle the potent chemotherapies they hit me with during the last five months.

Although, it was a tough decision at the time, it sounded great to me. Plan B would allow me to enjoy time with my family and make lasting memories. I agreed and said if during Plan B a miracle happens or if I go into remission, then I would continue back onto my original plan to get a stem cell transplant. As I decided on Plan B, I also prayed every night and day for God to give me guidance.

During my daily blog (see Chapter 13), I explained my options and told everybody that I was in a win-win situation. If I had gone into remission and gotten the chance to have a stem cell transplant, then I won. If I had lived for 10 months, spent quality time with my family, and then passed; I too would have won and gone to Heaven. I asked my blog-followers if they agreed, and they did.

Decitabine is given for seven days and then the patient has about a seven day recovery. Then he or she would enjoy two weeks before the next treatment. I started my first Decitabine treatment close to home at the Outpatient Cancer Transfusion Center in Pinehurst. The staff of nurses and pharmacists offered to come in on Saturday and Sunday to open the transfusion center just for me so that I would not have to get admitted into the hospital. What a kind act. They did not want to admit me to the hospital just to get my transfusions. I am forever thankful to my cancer doctors and nurses at First Health Outpatient Cancer Center; thank you from the bottom of my heart.

Again I prayed daily for guidance from God and had no idea of what was going to happen. I ask you again, do you believe in miracles? Maybe after I explain a little bit more about my case you too will believe in miracles. As my family physician, Dan Matthews, explained, "you not only have AML, you have the toughest to treat AML you can possibly have with terrible prognosticators." "You not have MDS, you have a three way translocation." Dan also said, "You are going to make it though, because your faith is strong and you are a tough fighter." Thank you for believing in me Dan.

I next scheduled a visit with my Priest Father Ricardo Sanchez at Our Lady of the America's Catholic Church in Candor, North Carolina. I visited Father Ricardo to have him give me my last rights and to perform the anointing of the sick. Father Ricardo, Laura, and I were all crying, and I felt weak in the knees. He asked me many questions to determine if I blame God for my cancers or any of my sicknesses? I explained that I did not, and that I had always thought of these cancers as a blessing. I told him that my journey had given me time to think about my life, God, and even more.

I also told him that I had only prayed for guidance, and I that I knew suffering was part of my journey. He and I started crying again. After he finished with my requests, he started looking for a medal for me to wear during the rest of my journey. Then he looked for a crucifix to give me, and jumped on his secretary's desk to wrestle this crucifix down off of the wall. I was now laughing at how passionate he was to get this crucifix down. Father Ricardo then said, "Chris, let me get you a brand new one and bless it."

So, imagine this, after watching Father Ricardo struggle for what seemed to be eternity; he walked me to a closet where he had 30 boxed crucifixes. Laura and I looked at each other, perhaps wondering if this simple trip to the closet should have been his first course of action. I found myself pondering if he had been the one that was not thinking clearly due to too much chemotherapy. But, retrospectively I feel that Farther Ricardo was nervous because of all the emotions during our meeting.

That day with Father Ricardo was THE CHE-MOment on which I base this book. I felt like the good Lord removed the burden of worrying, and felt like the weight had been lifted off of my shoulders. God is great! From that day forward everything started clicking, and now I was a true believer in beating the odds that had been stacked against me.

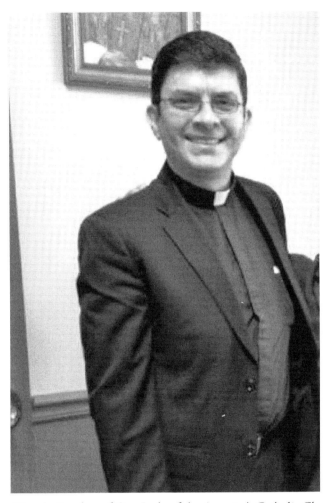

Father Ricardo Sanchez of Our Lady of the America's Catholic Church in Candor. My CHE-MOment with Father Ricardo F. Sanchez. Thank you for the gift of a second chance Lord! Thank you Father Ricardo for blessing me and giving me hope in miracles. I received the guidance that I prayed for and took the chance on the stem cell transplant.

Following my visit with Father Ricardo, I felt like the world had been lifted off of my shoulders. The best way to explain my feelings is through lyrics from a Johnny Cash song, **Unchained**: "Oh, I am weak. Oh, I know I am vain. Take this weight from me, Let my spirit be unchained!" I played this song on my iPod many times during my journey and felt emotional. I felt closer to God that day and every day forward.

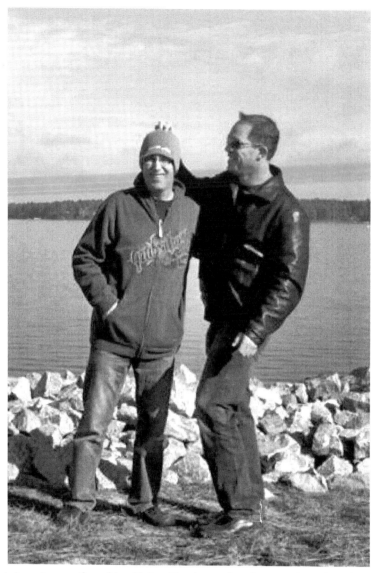

This is a picture of my friend Marc Tomberg when he visited me from Florida. Marc planned the visit because he knew things were getting tough, and that I was starting Plan B. Thank you for taking the time to visit Marc, that trip will always mean the world to me. I also had another friend travel from Florida, Dan Grose. Unfortunately I do not have a picture of him. Nevertheless, Dan's visit was great.

Dan, Laura and I went to breakfast and had a blast catching up on old times. Thank you Dan for also taking time out of your schedule to visit. I am so lucky to have great friends from grade school. Thank you.

Another great quotation to focus on during your travels:

"Miracles come in moments. Be ready and willing." Wayne Dye

Well, guess what happened after my first seven day treatment of Decitabine. I had to recover, and then I planned another trip with the family. We traveled up to Ridgefield, Connecticut to stay with my in-laws. We had a great time and I tried to get out as often as my body would allow. When I returned to Pinehurst, it was time for another bone marrow biopsy. I was really feeling great; maybe a miracle was starting to take shape? Maybe by releasing my fear and leaving the worrying to God was starting to work. Was this the miracle that my family and friends were praying for everyday.

The first of many miracles unfolded. My brother Billy came up as a perfect 10-for-10 match for transplanting his stem cells in me. WOW, you only have a 30% chance of having a sibling match. If your siblings are not matches, you have a 1 in 30,000 chance of having a match in the National Bone Marrow Registry. You see, I only have one sibling, so my chances were probably even lower than 30%. Billy was a PERFECT MATCH. What a gift, what a miracle! I now have renewed faith that my original plan had a great chance of happening. Never GIVE UP! Never GIVE UP! Thank you LORD.

While doing my Bone Marrow Biopsy, Dr. Moore and I had a great conversation about our Plan B. He asked what my blast levels would need to be for me to feel comfortable to move on to stem cell transplant. I knew through being a medical rep that you need less than or close to 5% blasts. Five percent blasts means that about 5% of all your cells are cancerous or pre-cancerous. Remember you need at least 10% blasts to be diagnosed with AML. I originally started at close to 30% blasts which is an aggressive form of AML. The transplant of my Brother's stem cells would serve as the fighter to kill the 5% cancer cells.

I next asked Dr. Moore what UNC would need me to be at to move on to stem cell transplant. He stated 5% or less. I told Dr. Moore my goal was 2%. He explained that Decitabine has a track record of lowering blast levels by less than 50%, meaning that I had a chance of going from 12%

to 6%, and that my goal of 2% might be a little too lofty. Dr. Moore then mentioned that my blast levels could also go up slowly with Decitabine or stay steady. Remember that Decitabine is meant to prolong life and not meant to work as a cure. I then told Dr. Moore that something is different now. I felt so damn good. I felt as if a miracle is taking place. He smiled and said, "I pray and hope so Chris."

I talked with Laura and said that I would go to stem cell transplant if my blasts get down to 2%. Laura questioned why I expected to get that low given that I had not gone below 12%. I told her that I was feeling the best I had in 10 months and I felt that something great was going to happen.

Wow, something beyond GREAT happened! My phone rang, and it was late on a Friday. Dr. Moore was on the phone line trying to hold himself together. "Chris, are you sitting down?" I explained that I was not. Dr. Moore then said, "Chris your are not going to believe this. What do you think your blasts are?" I replied that I felt great and believed that my blasts had come in at 5%. But, something told me that 2% was my number. Dr. Moore said, "I cannot believe this, your blast are at 2%!" I broke down crying, and so did he.

I could not believe that I prayed for guidance and received a sign in the form of 2% blasts. My answers came to me; it is now GO time Chris. My gut also told me that I had time to take another vacation. So we enjoyed some time with family again.

I came back in to do another bone marrow biopsy at UNC to see where my blasts were; just in case. My transplant coordinator Debbie started the ball rolling, and contacted my brother Billy to fly in and get checked out one more time before collection of his stem cells. By the way, I forgot to tell you that Billy hates going to the doctors or hospitals. He has a fear of needles and gets nervous when it comes to any treatment. He wanted to help me so bad. He said that this was his chance to save my life, and that this process was special to him. Billy constantly reminded me that this is how everything was meant to happen.

The great thing about collecting stem cells and or the bone marrow process is that it has become much easier on the donor. Doctors used to drill into the donor's bones in several places to remove the stem cells. Now, they have the donor administer Neupogen shots IM or Intramuscular into the belly fat/muscle. The donor has to do these shots for several days. This forces the stem cells to leave the marrow and move into the blood circulation. Neupogen shots are usually used with oncology patients to increase white blood cell count.

Next the donor gets hooked up to an aphaeresis machine to have blood collected out of one arm and delivered right back into the other arm. As the blood filters through the machine, the machine collects the stem cells out of circulation. The tough part is that process can take up to six hours, and the donor cannot move. If the donor has to use the restroom then they have to unhook the needles and then start over. Laura sat next to Billy the entire six hours feeding him, scratching his nose, and entertaining him with an Apple iPad.

My Brother had to fly in one more time to have his collection. To keep stress levels low, I opted to have Billy's stem cells frozen. That way there would not be any issues with trying to organize the collection and the stem cell transplant in the same day. I also asked UNC if they could remove more stem cells than are needed. This way if I needed any additional stem cell transplants or if the cancer came back, I would have some frozen and ready. You see, the process gets complicated with trying to keep everything organized. Freezing the stem cells does not affect the potency or the effectiveness of the stem cells, so why not make it easier on everybody involved.

Billy flew in to Raleigh Durham, and Laura picked him up in the morning. I was now being admitted back into the hospital, this time for a total of 100 days, which included a stay at the SECU House. I was in surgery getting another port installed, this time on the left side of my chest. I was a mess but a hematologist's dream with two ports and ready to roll.

A stem cell transplant is a big decision to make, and many patients decide against doing their transplant. Patients mainly decide this because it truly is one of the toughest procedures to endure. Receiving another person's cells and making the body ready for this foreign matter is an involved and delicate procedure. This is the risk that many people will take on to gain further life.

Well, I was now ready and willing to continue on my journey. God gave me my guidance of 2% blasts and I knew it was GO TIME! Dr. Serody told me that this would be the toughest thing I would ever do in my life. I commented back to Dr. Serody, "What do you mean; my three surgeries, thyroid ablation, six and a half weeks of head and neck radiation, and seven months of chemotherapy was not the toughest thing I ever endured?" Dr. Serody laughed and said, "Believe it or not, this will be tougher than what you have been through." He also said, "Chris I have faith in you and know you can do it." Dr. Serody also mentioned several times that this was the only way you could beat your forms of AML and MDS. I looked at Dr. Serody and Debbie my transplant coordinator in the eyes, and said, "get the photographer ready because I am going to be the next success story of this hospital." The disease needed more hope and guidance surrounding it.

"A strong positive mental attitude will create more miracles than any wonder drug."—Patricia Neal

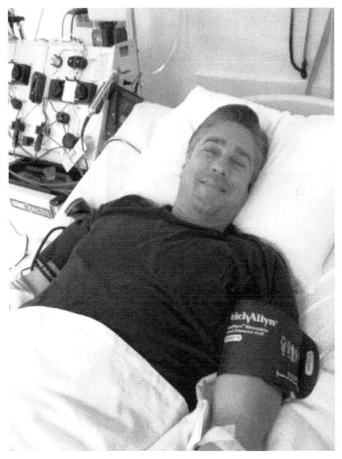

My awesome brother Billy delivering my "NEW LIFE" to UNC Cancer Hospital. Thank you Billy; you mean the world to me. You can see how he has both arms connected to the aphaeresis machine. Alicia was Billy's Bone Marrow Coordinator. Thank you Alicia for doing such a great job with Billy.

CHAPTER 9

STEM CELL TRANSPLANT
AND MY NEW BIRTHDAY

"The doors we open and close each day decide the lives we live."
Flora Whittemore

So true—what a quotation. If I did not choose to open the door and get my transplant, my days on earth would have been over for sure. Remember I was on Plan B, and that was only going to prolong my life for up to 10 months. Thank you Lord, for giving me the guidance and delivering a miracle!

Let me share one more crazy story before I get into the meat of the transplant and the rest of my venture. Before my brother Billy was flying up to UNC to deliver his cells, I was pondering second thoughts. My second thoughts were coming from other patients warning me to be prepared for a difficult and risky transplant experience.

Even though God gave me the signs that I prayed for, I was still scared out of my damn mind. Was I ready for another all-out war against cancer? Did I have enough in the tank? How would this affect my family? How will I afford all the medical bills? Believe me, these questions and doubts will hit you like a ton of bricks, and trust me that your guidance will come through prayer. Clearly, this was going to be a difficult and painful process. And, there were not guarantees of success; I was still quite aware of the possibilities of my own demise.

I freaked out so much that I called my Brother just before he was getting on his plane. I told him that I was wigging out and instead of going to the hospital to deliver his cells that I wanted to go Cheesecake Factory for lunch. Billy laughed and said, "You are out of your mind . . . ." I think my main problem was not wanting to put everybody through more pain and worry. I also did not want to put Billy through the hassle of getting hooked up to the apheresis machine. The fact that needles and doctors freak Billy out worried me too. I, like anyone in my situation, was having second thoughts; a bit of buyer's remorse if you will. Chances are, you too may have second, third, and forth thoughts. After all, these are huge decisions made under tremendous anxiety.

Just the price of admission alone scared the hell out of me. They call transplant plant patients million-dollar patients. The cost to insurance companies for a transplant runs anywhere from $1,000,000 to $2,000,000. That includes the cost of all the chemotherapies, the transplant, and the one year after-care or post-transplant care. Each time they do a bone marrow biopsy on you, the hospital pockets anywhere from $5,000 to $8,000. No doubt about it, cancer is big business, profitable, and expensive to treat.

Well, my brother Billy slapped some sense in to me and said that we were not going to Cheesecake Factory. Billy said, "I am going to give my cells today and you are going to let me continue on my part of our journey." He also said, "I know this is the right thing for you, and I know that you are going to walk away from this nasty disease." Billy, thank you for kicking me in the ass and keeping me straight.

Well, I rolled out of surgery and the fun began.

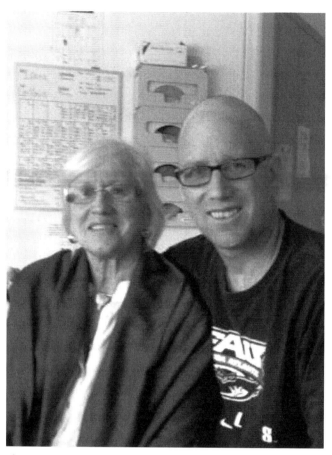

Picture of my wonderful and loving Mom. She stayed with me each day during my 35-day transplant. She said that she was my Eagle, flying above making sure that I was going to be safe and see my way through my 2 year trek. Wow, Mom you were a true inspiration of hope and healing during my transplant. THANK YOU from the bottom of my heart.

Mom's favorite quotation that she repeated often during my venture:

"Yesterday is history. Tomorrow is a mystery. Today is a gift. That's why it's called the present." ~ Eleanor Roosevelt

This next picture was taken during my last climb before my cancers hit. I feel that it is a great time to show you a photo of me during a perfect day of climbing with my friend Aaron. The day was beautiful, and the temperature was 46 degrees. I remember every detail about this day because I used this day as one of my visuals of a normal life again.

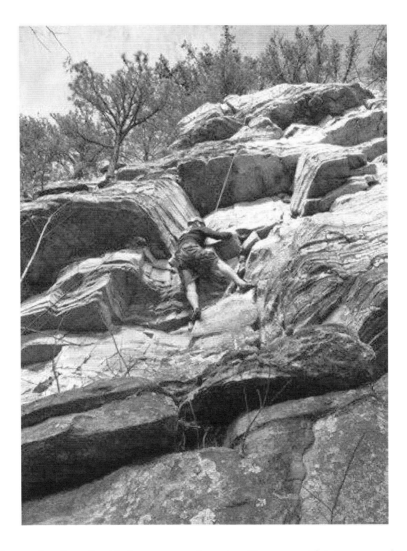

Remember how I said that you need to visualize yourself doing something that relaxes you and brings you to a state of being centered. This is something I practiced in my mind every day during my travels.

Make sure that you have an iPod or MP3 player with your favorite music. A great way to relax is deep breathing, visualizing activities that you enjoy, and listening to your favorite music. I even added many Zen songs to my iPod to get me into a state of relaxation.

You have probably heard the saying no pain-no gain? Well with every disease you are going to experience some sort of pain and suffering. I understand that I often express this in my book, and I truly believe that pleasure and appreciation in life is always rewarded after pain and suffering is experienced.

With my new port taking hold, my treatments began hot and heavy. This three-pronged Hickman port would also serve as the access to deliver Billy's cells. The medication parade also started on day one, as well as, several days of the heaviest chemo I would receive to date.

They put me on 15 plus medications. Each medication would protect me against threats that could come up during transplant. They placed me on an anti-rejection medication called Prograf. All transplant patients have to go on Prograf or one of the many anti-rejection medications available. No matter what the transplant is for, anti-rejection medication is needed to ensure that your immune system system does not attack the new cells or new organ.

They also put you on an anti-viral medication called Valtrex, an anti-fungal medication Diflucan, another anti-fungal called Voriconazole, steroid medications such as Prednisone, Actigall to protect the liver, Norvasc to treat high blood pressure caused by Prograf, Prilosec to protect the stomach, Magnesium to replace what is depleted from Prograf, Zofran to keep nausea at bay, and Ativan to help with sleep. That is just the start of the medication circus throughout your transplant.

The tough situation for me and for everybody on the transplant floor was getting sleep, especially the first five nights. All hospitals are loud. Moreover, if you add steroids and Prograf to the mix, sleep becomes virtually impossible. Do not forget your earplugs; you are going to need them.

While I am on the topic of items that you will need for transplant or hospital stays, the following is a list of the most important items; soft toilet paper, earplugs, iPod or radio, laptop computer, walking clothes, toe nail clippers, electric razor, comfortable pajamas, sweat pants, t-shirts, tennis shoes for walking, cotton only undergarments, laundry soap, movies or DVDs, puzzles, books, magazines, deck of cards, and anything else that may be your favorite indoor hobby. I hope that this helps you, and that it prevents your caregiver from making multiple trips.

The next thing I am going to share with you is something that the doctors will not tell you beforehand. This is something that took me for a ride that I will never forget. I now know what people experienced in the 1960s with mind expanding drugs. I also understand why medical professionals utilized steroids to induce psychosis in mental hospitals years ago. Another issue that added to the fun was that I did not sleep the first five days, which only increased my steroid side effects.

This experience that I speak of hit me on my fifth night around 1:00am. Suddenly the room started coming alive! On the wall there were three sizes of blue gloves in boxes. The gloves were coming alive as wicked mean cats with huge claws. I still remember it like yesterday. I then tried to clear my head, but that was going to be impossible because of sleep deprivation. I then turned my attention to my Dots candy box in my room, but that was a huge mistake. The colors on a Dots candy box are vibrant and this only added to my far from earth event.

The Dots were turning into dragons spitting fire! Shit, is this really happening to me? Pinch, pinch—yes sir this shit is happening and not stopping anytime soon. Of course while I am experiencing this, I did not dare call anyone. There is no way in hell that they will believe me. I finally fell asleep around 4:00am, and woke up in the morning to my usually blood work and medications.

The next event is what really pissed me off. I waited for the gang of doctors and interns to march through at their usually time of grand rounds. This is what I meant by the doctors will never tell you the whole truth; if they did, nobody would put themselves through a transplant. I brought up my experience from the night before and told them that I had never done any hardcore drugs in my life. They laughed and said that this was the first time they had heard this—LIARS! What they forget, is that smart patients talk to other transplant patients on the floor and know the truth.

I talked to my neighbor and asked him if he experienced anything crazy during his first several nights. Right away, he said that he had hallucinations and felt depressed. He said that the doctors made him feel like he should go on antidepressants. I gave him a high five and said I knew the doctors were lying to me; for good reason of course. I told him that I experienced the same things. Do you blame the doctors from lying? This is a serious investment in getting their patients through this procedure. If we knew the truth, we might be hesitant on going through with the transplant.

Just another day at the office, LOL. I constantly joked around with the doctors stating that if I was not there the next day, to not come looking for me. I asked them for plenty of sheets because I was going to start tying them together to make a ladder or rope to escape that joint. All kidding aside, I knew that I had to hold it together to accomplish what we were all trying to obtain; the extended gift of life.

Although I was losing sleep and things were not getting any better, I still focused on what I wanted to do when I was better. I listened to my iPod for hours focusing on my breathing. I prayed for continued guidance from God and my guardian angels. My favorite nurse "Sergeant" Barbara also kept me in line. She was great at her job and knew her stuff. We had our arguments. Nonetheless, Barbara was by far the most knowledgeable and the most focused nurse on the BMT Floor. Thank you for your great care Barbara.

During all of this craziness, my transplant day was only a couple of days away. I was buzzing with excitement, and at the same time, I was scared out of my mind. Once I took on my Brother's cells there was going to be no turning back.

Even though I was not getting sleep and I was starting to get depressed, I still exercised every day and never missed. My goal was to exceed a marathon in the 30-day transplant stay. The BMT unit had a program for patients that exceeded a marathon in 30 days. This seems like a ton of walking for someone undergoing the most brutal chemo that any cancer patient has to endure. Nonetheless, it is less than a mile per day. You can DO IT! Please walk or exercise every day and I promise that it will make your comeback that much easier. They call your transplant day "day zero" and then the calendar starts at day one post-transplant from there. Around day seven, the chemo starts to kick your butt. So be ready for a fight and enjoy your transplant day.

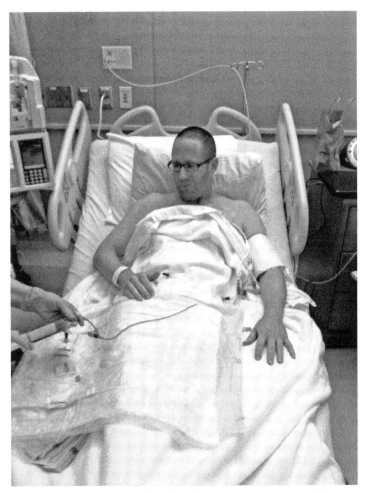

Here is a picture of my "new birthday" or day zero. You can see Barbara inserting Billy's cells into my port one tube at a time. I received 13 tubes of Billy's stem cells. I later learned that my "New Birthday" was the same birthday as my late Nana (May 14th). Wow, I know that Nana was looking down on me with a big smile.

This was it, my big day was here. My pilgrimage started on 11/11/11 when I was diagnosed with AML and I received my transplant on 05/14/12. The reason I emphasize this, is that it may take you a long time to get there, but the trip is worth the price of admission. Just to think that I was contemplating Plan B or going to the Cheesecake Factory just a couple of months before my transplant day.

I will tell you now that you should enjoy your day zero and your transplant day because it is like watching paint dry. The day is laid back and they give you the medication needed to fight anything that may come your way. If your cells were frozen like mine, the chemical that they use is DMSO. Well, DSMO has the tendency to smell up the room, and the smell lasts for about three days. The nurses explained the smell to be like creamed corn or tomato soup. The patient cannot smell it, but everybody else can. They ask you to suck on peppermints during the actual transplant. Next, Barbara asked me, "are you ready for the first tube of your Brother's cells?" I said heck yes, even though I was nervous as all get out. As the first tube was attached to my port and started to enter my chest, I felt this surge of energy or rush. WOW! This feeling was incredible—I cannot explain it though. This surge of energy then turned to a heat in my body and my skin started flushing around my chest. I knew at that moment that this was meant to be and this was what God wanted for me. Each tube gave me the same sensation and the same surge of energy.

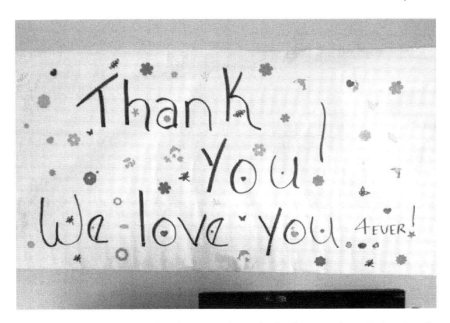

This picture above was a Thank You card to Billy for flying in from Delray Beach to deliver his stem cells to UNC. The process was stressful for Billy and I thank him and Joseph from the bottom of my heart. Billy, there is no doubt about it, you saved my life! I am forever indebted to you and Joseph for being so giving.

I took on the tenth tube, and I had this feeling of being full. That was weird because the tubes were going into my blood circulation and not into my stomach. I continued to feel full and uncomfortable and asked if this would pass soon. Barbara said, "absolutely." I definitely worried about this day, but please do not waste your energy worrying before you get there. Like I said, enjoy your day zero to day six because you definitely will feel the wrath of the chemo catch-up to you.

I called my Brother to let him know that he was losing his *"MOJO baby,"* just like in the *Austin Powers movie, The Spy who Shagged Me.* Billy laughed it off and said, "I have plenty of MOJO to go around." Thank you Billy for loving me so much and giving your stem cells, which definitely comes with the risks and your share of pain. Love you forever Billy!

My next few days would be uneventful, and I would eat as much as I could. Please eat as much as you can, because when the chemo side effects hit you, your appetite will quickly leave. Now, if a patient receives his or her own cells, the comeback is quick. This is in contrast to an allogeneic transplant when the patient receives someone else's cells. If the patient receives someone else's cells, the comeback can take up to two years or more.

My plan was to be back at work around the one year mark, post-transplant. It is always good to set realistic goals for yourself. I always set goals because it kept my mind from focusing on the negative. Goals also kept me on track, so that I would not get depressed and doubt my comeback. **"If you want to live a happy life, tie it to a goal, not to people or things."**—Albert Einstein

My choice of food during day zero through day six was salmon. Grilled salmon was perfect and a healthy choice. As you already know, you have to force yourself to eat during your venture. I knew when the chemo hit that I was going to feel the wrath. That was an understatement, and I thought I was ready for anything. I had already taken on so many chemo treatments that I knew I could hang with this one. Well, that is where I was wrong. This was a chemo with many extra weapons tied in that had a powerful side effect profile. Do not worry. You too will take on the challenge and feel better before you know it.

My doctors did warn me that I should get ready for about seven to ten days of serious pain. The chemo regimen that they give you mainly hits your gastrointestinal (GI) tract. The whole entire GI tract is affected. It starts in your mouth with sores and goes all the way through to your butt. This is where the soft toilet paper will help you. The hospital supplies toilet paper that compares to sand paper.

Now, do not freak out because I had head and neck radiation, which already had my mouth raw and vulnerable. So as you could imagine the pain was intense. The sores in my mouth were dime size, and were on FIRE for 10 days. I never took pain killers during my journey, except for my tonsillectomy and for this part of my tour. I marched through all the pain killers, and finally settled on Fentanyl intravenously. This is the strongest and most potent narcotic out there. The pain was so intense that they gave me a pain pump and a button to deliver as much Fentanyl that I needed. I never worried about getting hooked because I knew this would only last six to seven days. If you have an addictive personality, please be careful on how many days or the type of narcotics that your doctors chose for you. Please remember to be your own advocate.

While you are in the hospital for your 35-day transplant stay, please be sure to have everybody scrub their hands before they come in your room and before they leave your room. Also have your caregiver (Spouse, Mom, Dad, Son or Daughter) sterilize the room with antibacterial wipes. This will make certain that you keep your room as germ free as possible. The reason I say this is that once Clostridium difficile (C-diff) or Vancomycin-resistant Enterococcus (VRE) starts spreading from person to person, the only way to beat it is to keep vigilant on cleaning the room. Cleaning hands and luck helps too. If VRE or C-diff spreads throughout the hospital and passes on to you, this could mean a much tougher comeback than anticipated. VRE and C-diff are devastating to your GI tract and cause loose stools. Not exactly what a leukemia or cancer patient needs, more weight loss and more pain.

If you keep a clean room and make sure everyone washes his or her hands, then you are well on your way to avoiding these nasty bugs. I am speaking from experience because I was able to avoid it due to being an advocate for myself. I always put limits on the amount of traffic in and out of my room, and I would also put on a pair of gloves and help keep the room sanitized.

The patients that had VRE and C-diff had to wear coats and protection over their bodies while they exercised or anytime they came out into the hallway. Please take the time and protect yourself from germs, fungus, shingles, etc. Once you do chemotherapy, your immune system is shot for three weeks time, and it is up to you to avoid these possible issues. Do not forget to wear your mask in the hallways and out in public. You can also ask other people that come in your room to wear masks, and if it is FLU season, you can never be cautious enough. Have your caregiver sterilize the phone, your bed rails, your TV remote, and all other items that the cleaning crew does not focus on much.

When you are neutropenic, be sure to bathe each day, use moisturizer to prevent cracks in your skin, utilize a foam toothbrush, do not use dental floss, and do not scratch any cuts or insect bites. Remember that your immune system is basically ineffective and cannot protect you when you are neutropenic. The reason for this is that chemotherapy targets good cells as well as bad cells. Guess what the good cells do? They are your immune system, and they fight infections and disease. So, please be vigilant in protecting your health, especially in the hospital. A hospital is best described as a petri dish with windows, walls, and doors.

I believe I mentioned that I was emotional during my 35-day transplant stay. My walking partner Ricky that I spoke about in earlier chapters was not doing well. When I received my transplant, Ricky was getting sick. He was hit with VRE, C-diff, a mold infection in the sinuses, and bacteria in his blood. I was able to talk to Ricky, however, there was not much reply because of his condition. During my exercise time, when I walked around the BMT unit, I would pass by Ricky's room. I could not do a lap without tearing-up. I still cry to this day when I think about Ricky.

Ricky was my pace car, and he was my friend that I made on 4-Onc. I prayed endlessly that Ricky would pull out of this, and that his transplant would take hold. I also prayed that his Brother's cells would overcome all of this. Laura and I also talked to his wife Joni and his son Austin. I remember buying golfing and sports magazines for his birthday. He was a huge UNC basketball fan and loved to play golf. I heard that he was a great player, and I knew he was an awesome person.

Unfortunately, Ricky did not make it. He passed on during my transplant. I was lucky to know Ricky, and I am a better person because of him. He was such a fighter, and he was the champion walker during our several months at UNC. Thank you for being my friend Ricky. I know you are swinging your golf clubs up in heaven and enjoying being with God.

CHAPTER 10

MY CLOSING DAYS ON THE BONE MARROW TRANSPLANT FLOOR

My final week on the BMT floor was the hardest, because I could not wait to get out of the hospital. I was in UNC Hospital for a total of 116 days during my two-year trek. Total time in hospitals for all four of my cancers was close to 150 days in two years. Wow, what a JOURNEY! Remember that we are meant to go through this, and hopefully we learn our lessons during our down time—I know I have. Yes, I did cry on my last days before leaving the BMT. I guess you can blame the medications or the fact that I am Italian.

I learned my lessons, and now feel as if I need to pay it forward. That is how this book came together. This is part of my plan to help people get through their battle; whatever their battle may be.

I also wanted to talk to you about food and eating because it becomes difficult to eat with no appetite and lack of taste. If you do have an appetite after chemo treatments, usually you are battling your taste buds. That is one side effect that can take months to straighten out. Try adding head and neck radiation to the mix. I still to this day cannot taste chocolate, and sometimes after radiation, it could take two to three years to get your normal tastes back.

I lost a total of 60 pounds during my treatments, and you to will lose your fair share of weight. My best piece of advice is to listen to your doctors. Also listen to your own body; your cravings will tell you what you want. If you can do sweets, find a milkshake you can drink and do many of them. Even though I could not taste dairy, I still found that mint milkshakes worked for me. They were tough to get down, but you need to get nutrition, or your body will not be strong enough to comeback.

Most medical professionals will tell you to stay away from sugar because it can be a food source for cancer. However, during my comebacks, I looked at the overall picture. I did try to keep sugar at the minimum. Nonetheless, my body craved milkshakes, smoothies, and donuts. The tough thing that the medical professionals do not understand is that we have a lack of taste and sometimes we have to eat sweet items early on in our comebacks.

Eating is essential, and when you can eat, DO IT! These are definitely just suggestions and your nutritionist and doctors have much say in your diet. I just wanted to touch upon what worked for me and hoped that it would help you.

After I completed many of my chemotherapies, my numbers were close to zero, if not zero. I ate steak to help boost my platelets; I ate salmon to boost my omega, etc. I also ate tons of asparagus on the grill. Asparagus has many beneficial attributes that help chemotherapy patients. Read up on the benefits on the Internet, and I think you will be surprised.

Please do not let the nutritionists quilt you into drinking those terrible protein shakes or juice boxes unless you enjoy the taste. Of course, if you can get them down and you like them, please feel free to drink them; they are great for you.

Even though I had a tough time getting down smoothies, I still forced them down because of the fruits that my body needed. If you want to beat your cancers, you must EAT. Please do your best to keep your weight up during your journey. Once your comeback is behind you, you must change your ways and adapt your diet to help keep your body cancer free.

Some say once you beat your cancer that vegan is a top choice. Although, you do not have to go to that extreme unless you want to of course. During my comeback, I ate whatever I wanted, and I also ate whatever I felt was the right thing for me. I ate steak, milkshakes, high protein meals, salmon, sea bass, smoothies loaded with fresh blueberries, strawberries, oranges, etc.

Please remember that my suggestions are only my suggestions from being a two-year cancer fighter and from being in the medical industry for 10 years. I only want to make your comeback quicker, your chemotherapies take hold better, and get you the right nutrients for your body to give you the best chance to make cancer your ally.

When you complete your comeback and want to keep getting good results at your monthly and yearly visits, please be as healthy as you can. My freezer and fridge is full of veggies and fruits. If I am out and the kids want to eat at Subway, I simply order all veggies on a whole wheat sub roll with oil and vinegar. Try it. It is great! You can eat healthy almost anywhere. I knew I had to change my ways because of the fact that my body produced four different types of deadly cancer. This is a great time to bring up the foods that increase the chance of cancer as referenced by _http://www.Naturalnews.com_. They list the following top ten food: genetically modified organisms, processed meats, microwave popcorn (bag linings), soda pop, diet beverages, refined white flours, refined sugars, dirty fruits (strawberries and grapes), farmed salmon and hydrogenated oils (used in processed foods.)

You either wake-up when the alarm goes off or you keep hitting the snooze button. Next, let me share this story with you. I knew this doctor that worked at an office in North Carolina during my career. I really looked up to this person. He was humble and always had time for me when I called on him. I was unaware that he was sick, and he hid his signs of being sick from everyone. He and I had many things in common; more in common that I would ever imagine.

This doctor was fighting a form of acute leukemia and had already tried everything. I guess one day he just realized that he wanted to live a normal life and did not want to take on treatments. This doctor did not tell anyone he was fighting this disease, not even his partners or friends. He was divorced; therefore, it was easier to hide. The only reason I knew this doctor had leukemia was that he passed-on right there at work during a lunch and learn. Everybody was floored. I could not believe that he hid this and looked completely normal.

The reason I bring this up is that there will come a time in your treatments that you too will want to live a normal life again. Please fight the urge. This doctor ignored his journey and stopped fighting his disease.

He just wanted to be normal. Well, as you see, acute leukemia is a deadly disease and will catch up with you quickly. I wish I knew this doctor was going through this so that I could have spent more time with him.

My hope while writing this book was to think about every situation that may come up during your journey. I want your journey to be successful. I want you to have the best chance at beating the odds. Never give up hope. I will never give up hope, and I will always fight no matter what.

I also want to share with you what *Tarascon Pocket Oncologica* says about AML so that you do not get caught up in statistics and odds. What you have to realize is that these are just statistics. You do not have to be part of the statistics—this is your venture. If you are diagnosed with AML and your cytogenetics are poor, the statistics say that your chance of survival past five years is 5% to 12%. This means that I have a 12% chance of living past five years. Terrible odds, right? There is no doubt I will blow past five years and live a normal life 30 years from now. These are just statistics and not today's statistics. Everybody is different too! Please strive to have the same attitude and stay off of the Internet the best you can.

See, you cannot let statistics or odds get you down. If your AML is less severe and your cytogenetics are good, then your odds go up to a 60% chance of making it to five years or more. These are just numbers and you have to add in age, overall health before cancer, and many other factors. I hope that this all makes sense?

Please do not get caught up reading stuff on the Internet. Keep your chin up, and focus on what you will be doing in your new life once you walk out the doors of the cancer hospital. *Tarascon Pocket Oncologica* also says the risk factors that increase your chances of being diagnosed with AML are: ionizing radiation, occupational benzene, petrochemical, paint or pesticide exposure, chemotherapy with alkylating agents, and anti-psoriasis agents.

Well, speaking about walking out the doors of the hospital, it was now my turn to walk out and check into the SECU House. UNC and all cancer hospitals make you stay within 30 miles of your post-transplant care. They will ask you stay until day100. My home was 75 miles from the hospital, so I had to find a place to stay while making my comeback from the transplant. The SECU House was perfect. The SECU House charged $50 a night, and the great thing was that most insurances reimburse you for your cost of up to $100 per night.

I want to end this chapter with a great quotation that helped me many times: **"Courage is being afraid but going on anyhow."** ~Dan Rather

CHAPTER 11

SECU HOUSE AND POST-TRANSPLANT CARE

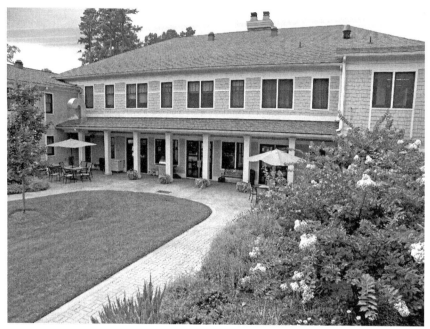

The SECU House in Chapel Hill. What a great treat to have this awesome facility available to cancer patients that live to far from UNC Hospital.

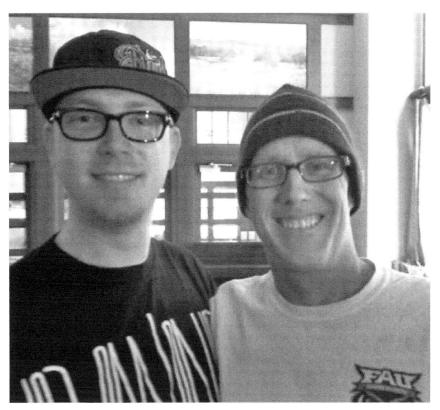

This is a picture of my Caregiver/Brother-in-law Adam Smith at The SECU House. Thank you for taking care of me during the 65 days at The SECU House Adam. I am lucky to have you as a Brother-in-law. Thank you again for everything Adam. Love you Brother.

"I made up my mind not to care so much about the destination, and simply enjoy the journey." What a great quotation by David Archuleta.

The reason why I like this quotation so much is that it reflects my *CHE-MOment* when God answered my prayers. We as humans always want to know how things are going to turn out during most situations; however, in many cases it is more appropriate to experience the trip.

It took me many months to realize that I should leave the worrying to God, and then to my surprise the burden was lifted from my shoulders. We must care less about the destination and let the journey play out. I guess what I am saying is that you must trust in God and your guardian angels more than ever have in your life. No matter what happens, it is better to go through your tour with less stress and less burden. Your chances significantly increase when you relax and meditate during your campaign. **"If God is your partner, make your plans BIG!"** —D.L. Moody

Wow, I finally made it to The SECU House. I visualized this during my transplant. I could not wait to get to this point, because I knew that I was in the home stretch. Do not get me wrong, this was also a tough and painful part of the venture. The reason why I say this is acute GVH is prevalent during the first few months after transplant.

GVH is a reactionary response that the body gives off while your new stem cells are trying to graft or take hold. This is your body protecting its home turf while the new organ or new stem cells are trying to make a home. The doctors help your body calm down a bit with a drug called Prograf, which is an immunosuppressant. This drug interrupts your immune system so that it does not attack the new stem cells.

My GVH came in the form of skin rashes, large joint arthritis, and severe stomach cramping. My doctors fought the GVH by increasing my Prograf which made me tired. I also could not exercise for the first time during my pilgrimage. When I tried to exercise, my joints ached, and my muscles became sore. I relaxed during the next couple of months and focused on eating and gaining weight. I came out of transplant weighing 152. I had lost a total of 40 pounds during my transplant.

My days at The SECU House consisted of sleeping and eating. The great thing was that Adam loved to eat also. Early on we cooked steaks on the grill to get my platelets up. I could not taste much, but I knew I had to gain weight. Adam and I frequented Carrabba's, Chinese food, Panera, Merritt's, and Mexican food. Merritt's was known for its BLTs, and Merritt's has been around since 1929. They fly in their tomatoes if it is off season, and they bake their own bread. This was by far the best BLT I have ever had, and now I know why they are world-famous. I will never forget that the owner asked if I was fighting cancer, and she also asked if she could pray with me. Wow, a complete stranger prayed with me, and she was so sincere that she made me cry. Each time I go to UNC for my appointments, I now go to Merritt's for lunch. I am a customer for life.

Adam helped me with all of my medications and put steroid cream on my back to keep the GVH at bay. I was having to go to UNC three times a week for routine post-transplant care. Adam and I rode the bus system which worked out great. We attended my appointments in the morning and then ate lunch on Franklin Street after the appointments.

We spent most of our time watching movies that Adam brought with him from Connecticut. We also watched *Netflix*, and we cheered on the Miami Heat to their second World Championship. I was so relieved that LeBron James proved all those naysayers wrong. I am also a huge Marlins, Red Sox, Dolphins, Panthers, and FAU Owls fan.

During our time at The SECU House, we had many visitors. Erin and Charlie get the prize. They drove from Chicago to Georgia to drop off the kids and then up to Chapel Hill to visit me. They brought a blanket for me which was knitted by All Saints Lutheran Church in Blairsville, Georgia. Each stitch was made with a prayer. The blanket with a tag attached to it which read, "May God wrap you in the warmth of his love and the prayer of His Healing Hands always."

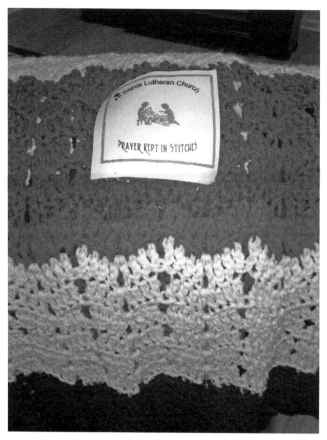

This is a picture of the blanket that Charlie and Erin brought me. I cannot tell you how much that meant to me. Thank you so much Erin and Charlie for your kind act. I needed that visit badly. I was having one of those dark days, and the blanket brought me back to feeling good.

Family support and love are so important during your journey. I forgot to mention earlier in my book that you should always welcome as much interaction with people through a blog, visits when your numbers are up, or phone calls. It is so easy to stay closed or wrapped up in your tour of duty that you do not allow people to communicate with you. That is why I connected through Carepages. I felt that if I kept everyone updated, they would appreciate being in the loop. This also helps with keeping the burden off of family members to receive too many phone calls, etc. Please be sure to allow people to follow and support you during your campaign.

People just want to be considerate and show their love for you; so please let them.

When it comes to the post-transplant care, most of the follow-up is to replace what is missing in your blood including electrolytes. Most of you already know that chemotherapy depletes your platelets, white blood cells (WBC), hematocrit (HMT) and absolute neutrophil count (ANC). Chemo also affects your magnesium levels, calcium levels, hair, skin, and of course your thinking. That is right, chemo brain is for real. Your processing becomes cloudy, and it becomes hard to concentrate on more than one thing.

Anyone going through a transplant will have low magnesium and potassium levels. Not just chemo affects your electrolytes. Prograf will deplete them also. The reason I bring this up is that most doctors will order magnesium and potassium to be given to you as a transfusion; more money for the hospital of course. If you are making trips back to hospital or transfusion center just for electrolytes, please ask for a supplement or tablet that you can take at home. You can buy 400mg magnesium oxide supplements at any pharmacy, and it sure beats getting extra transfusions. Keep in mind, you will need a prescription for the potassium tablets.

Always ask your doctor if any treatment comes in any other form or option. The last thing you want is to be hanging out in the hospital or transfusion center longer than needed. The remainder of the post-transplant care comes down to GVH, transfusions, checking blood, checking electrolyte counts, and bone marrow biopsies. You are also busy with running to the pharmacy because of the weekly medication tweaks. The transplant process is a fine balance between medicine and how the body reacts to the medicine and your new cells.

Before I forget, I wanted to share some more great memories during my stay at The SECU House. Below is a picture of Riley celebrating his 16th birthday—what a treat that was for me to see.

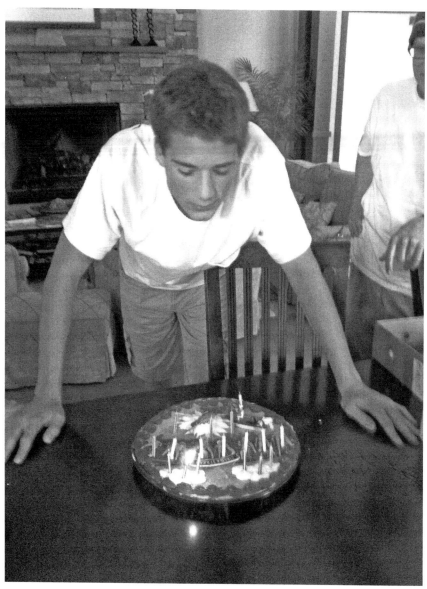

Happy 16th birthday Riley. My boy's are my light and mean so much to me. I love you guys. Thank you for all the memories and love over the last 16 years Riley and Brennan. You both are and will always be my inspiration!

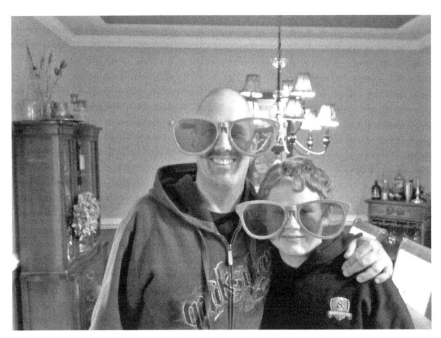

This is one of my favorite pictures during my two-year journey. We enjoyed a day of bowling and playing video games in the arcade. We won these glasses with our tickets from the arcade. Brennan and Riley always brought sunshine to me during my two years. We laughed and laughed at our photo that day. Thank you to all of my family for your love and support.

Another great memory was from the day I had a wild hair and wanted to go test drive a Porsche 911 Carrera S. Adam has a passion for race cars, and I knew this would be something that Adam would enjoy. I mentioned it to Adam, and he asked how the heck we were going to get the dealership to allow us to test drive a $125,000 car. I told Adam to not worry about that part. Adam was excited, and his interest in Porsche was just as strong as mine.

We headed up to the dealership and caught them on a slow day. We both walked around the car dealership in admiration. I met the General Manager and explained that we wanted to test drive the 911 Carrera S. "No problem", he explained, "just give me your driver license and I will make a copy." They pulled up a brand new 2013 911 Carrera S, and it was gorgeous. The sales person wanted to drive it with me first, and then pulled over to let me behind the wheel. I guess he did not know about chemo brain, and he trusted me to take over for him.

I first took the car on Interstate 40 and easily brought the speed up to 70 MPH. The sales guy then asked, "what are you waiting for? Punch it!" So I did. The 911 went from 70 to 125 plus MPH in a blink of an eye. Wow, our heads were pinned back from the g-forces. This was a great feeling and just what I needed that day.

Now, if I could only hit the lottery, I may be able to afford this masterful machine. Although, what is the old saying about the lottery; lotteries are a tax for people that are bad at math :))

This car handled like it was on rails—*Pretty Woman movie* quotation. I had so much fun that Adam and I went back the next day, so that Adam could take it for a test drive. Adam was even able to get the car up to speeds that I do not want to even type.

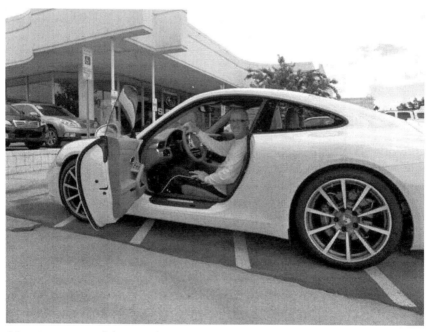

Here is a picture of the Porsche 911S that Adam and I test drove during our stay at the SECU House. What a RUSH!

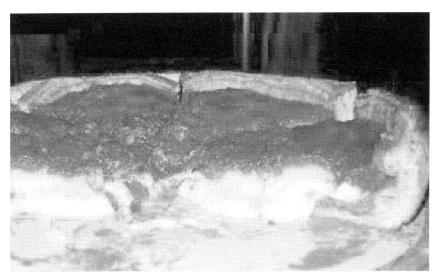

This pizza was another surprise that Adam and I received shortly after our Porsche experience. Charlie and Erin were so sweet and sent us two Giordano's Pizzas from Chicago. Laura, Riley, Brennan, Adam, and I enjoyed the heck out of that pizza. Wow, definitely one of the best pizzas in the Country. Erin and Charley-Thank you again for your generosity.

All great memories, but none were as wonderful as Adam spending two plus months with me to make sure that I get through my post-transplant care. I want to also thank my in-laws Ken and Cathe Smith for buying so many lunches and dinners that I lost count. Adam and I throughly enjoyed the meals. Although, Adam was not happy gaining the sympathy weight over the 65 plus days. It was fun while it lasted. The best part of coming back from chemotherapy is the guilt-free eating, which is enjoyable once you get some of your taste back.

While I am on the eating theme, let me talk a little on what foods are good after chemotherapy again. I am going to give you a list of what is best for coming back from chemo. Chemotherapy causes fatigue, mouth sores, lack of taste, and lack of nutrition. Since you cannot taste, much let me talk about the two most important foods after chemo. These are only my suggestions, so please clear anything you do through your doctors.

Steak or red meat is first on my list and many cancer websites too. Steak does many things for your body. Steak boosts platelets which is important for coming back from chemo. Steak will also help with sparing muscle tissue from being wasted, and steak is also a great source of protein. Of course, you need to talk to your doctors because there are special diets depending on your condition. There are diets to help renal function, heart function, liver function, etc. My best piece of advice I can give you is listen to your body and then clear foods through your doctor.

My second most sought after food is cooked asparagus. Let me list the benefits of asparagus: asparagus has been said to increase the effectiveness of chemotherapy, it helps fight chronic fatigue, it helps with constipation, it helps prevent bladder and urinary tract infections, it helps fight off high blood pressure, it can act as an anti-fungal and anti-viral, it is good for arthritis and joint pain, it is great for the heart, and it helps lower cholesterol. Should I list more or are you convinced? I know that the after effects are not that desirable with the smell in your urine. Nevertheless, the benefits definitely outweigh the stench. If you are prone to gout, asparagus may not be a good option for you. Again, please be sure to clear this with your healthcare professionals.

The following is a list of other recommendations: Bananas, yogurt, smoothies, cooked broccoli, cooked salmon, canned pears, and canned peaches. These are great lists to start and if followed, your comebacks will be much quicker. Do not forget to exercise which is also important for everything listed.

Let me also discuss the foods that you should avoid after chemotherapy or while on Prograf after transplant. The following foods are not recommended: sharp cheddar cheese, feta cheese, blue cheese, brie cheese, sliced meats from deli, unwashed raw fruits, raw veggies including broccoli, raw nuts, unpasteurized milk, unpasteurized yogurt, unpasteurized juices, oysters, or raw seafood, etc. Also remember to ask for your steak, chicken, and fish to be cooked well-done during your comeback. It would be best to use your commonsense, and if the food can harbor bacteria and is not cooked well, then it is probably a bad idea to consume.

Lets get back to my SECU House tour. I will never forget what I am about to tell you, and I hope that most patients would never do this. While I was at the SECU House there were also five other stem cell transplant patients there. I was outside one day exercising and doing my best to stay healthy. To my surprise, there were two transplant patients smoking cigarettes. You have got to be kidding me! I was floored! Here are two patients that have had transplants, which meant that they had at least $1,000,000 to $2,000,000 invested in them, and this is how they repay the system or God or their donor.

How in the heck can you have such disregard for yourself and your support system by smoking? No respect! I feel like puking just thinking about it again. Please take care of your transplanted cells; if not for you, how about for your donor.

Getting back to more positive thoughts. Another visit that stood out in my mind was when my friend Aaron stopped in for the weekend. He brought his guitar, some movies, and some food. Aaron also brought me books to read throughout my two-year journey, which was thoughtful. Aaron and Adam played on their guitars, and we sang a little bit too. We watched many great movies and had many great laughs.

Another great thing about The SECU House was that they had guitar players/musicians come in once a week and play for the critically sick patients that stayed there. What great people to give their time and make our day a little bit brighter. Some great talent came through The SECU House, and I will never forget those awesome days. I really looked forward to the musicians, talking with the other patients, and the food that organizations would bring in for us during the week. There are so many wonderful people in this world, and God is ever so present.

My stay at The SECU House was great. However, I had not been home in over 95 plus days. I missed home badly. Just sleeping in my own bed and waking up somewhere familiar would be super again. UNC would not let me go home until my follow-up visits were once every two weeks. This way I could do some follow-up blood work in Pinehurst.

Eventually, I would get down to one visit every month. My suggestion to you is ask your family doctor if he or she can help with follow-up blood work and medications. This will help, especially if your cancer hospital is quite a drive.

I am now in month-nine from my transplant date, and I still have my port which makes things easier when it comes to checking counts every month. I also try to make as many appointments as possible with my local oncologist or doctor so that my co-pays and cost of visits are lower.

While I am thinking about money again, make sure you check into gap insurance when you apply for social security disability. Please understand COBRA Insurance only lasts 18 months, and if your pilgrimage lasts longer than that, then you must get six months of gap Insurance to get you to Medicare Part B.

This is important because if you do not apply for gap insurance during your first couple of months of being approved for social security disability, they will not allow you to receive gap insurance. This means that you will be uninsured for six months until Medicare Part B goes into effect. Now with ObamaCare, things may be different because the laws change in 2014. Be sure to have this conversation with your hospital social worker so that you do not get caught with your pants down. Hopefully you will be back at work before you reach the 18-month cutoff for COBRA insurance.

Have you ever heard this joke: How many doctors does it take to change a lightbulb? It depends on if the lightbulb has health insurance. I saw this many times during my treatments because of the fact that I had private insurance. This is not a dig on doctors because we all know that their money source is scarce and their reimbursable amounts have drastically been decreased over the years.

Another great joke by Henny Youngman is: "My doctor grabbed my wallet and said, cough!" Don't get me wrong, I have the upmost respect for my doctor's, and I am thankful for them saving my life. These jokes are just to lighten the mood of the book :))

Do not forget about The Bone Marrow Foundation *One to One fund*. This will help with getting you through many financial difficulties. My suggestion to you is to start a Facebook Page or Carepage to connect with friends and family when your journey starts.

I wanted to talk about other things to do while you are healing and being away from your family. You could stream movies on Netflix, read motivational books, write a blog, pick up a new hobby, or maybe be a mentor for other cancer patients.

During my post-transplant visits to the bone marrow clinic and 4-Onc; there were many nurses, doctors, and people that I want to thank. Thank you Dr. Richards, Dr. Serody, Dr. Armistead, Dr. Gabriel, Paula, Debbie, Martha, Natasha, Karen, Amber, Sandra, Barbara, Robin, Laura, Drew, Jason, Alesha, Alicia, Trish, Becca, Kristen, Kelly, Steve, and Sonja just to name a few. I also want to thank the staff at The SECU House for their hospitality and all the people that donated their time and food during my stay. There are many pictures in the back of the book of these nurses and doctors.

I could keep naming people throughout my two-year experience; although, I need to keep you healthy and motivated to beat your disease or take on your challenge. Please do not listen to the negative people out there, and do not believe all those bad things on the Internet. Use all of that energy to motivate yourself to prove everybody wrong.

"Those who discourage you from your dreams have most likely already abandoned their own." Unknown Author

CHAPTER 12

ANOTHER SURPRISE, ANOTHER GUARDIAN ANGEL EXPERIENCE, AND MY NEW LIFE

"Develop an attitude of gratitude and give thanks for everything that happens to you, knowing that every step forward is a step toward achieving something bigger and better than your current situation."
—Brian Tracy

I know that this quotation is tough to read while you are in the middle of your battle or during your difficult situation that you may be facing; nevertheless, it is a great quotation to keep in your back pocket. You see, I am a huge believer that our lives are already prewritten and that there is a plan for each of us. I am also a huge believer that every experience in our lives happens for a reason. I know this sounds cliché, and you often hear these things from many people. We just need to look at these moments in our lives as wake-up calls. What is wrong with always looking at the glass as half-full?

I chose this quotation for this chapter because it was fitting to this part of my journey. You see, as I checked out of The SECU House, I received another HUGE surprise the first day I returned home. Before I share this surprise with you, I want you to understand that nothing can make me waiver or nothing can shake my foundation. You see, I have survived, and I will continue to survive—and you will too.

As I unpacked my clothes on my first night back, my wife Laura of 20 years said that she wanted to discuss something with me. Now, this was at bedtime, and she completely took me off-guard. Understand that our marriage had been a struggle for the last three years; however, I had felt that this two-year journey had only made our marriage stronger. Well, I was wrong. Laura told me that she just could not do this anymore. She said, "I just do not feel the same way I used to about us." This break-up felt like the classic break-up line; "It is not you, it is me" scenario. Wow! I took a couple of deep breaths and said, "Laura I am shocked that you waited to tell me on my first night back. Nonetheless, I am fine with the way you feel, and nothing can rattle my cage. You have given me two beautiful and loving boys, and you took care of me during my sickest of days." What else could I ask for out of a marriage? Laura gave me 20 great years!

I also told Laura that the most important aspect of divorce was the kids. We made a promise that night to never fight in front of the boys and to make the divorce amicable. Well, we did make the divorce amicable, and the whole divorce cost $750 dollars in paper work and attorney's fees.

I had fought for Laura over the past three years, and I was not not going to make a fool of myself. Have you ever heard the saying that you can only change yourself, because to change another person requires the other person to accept change? I know that may be a mouth full. However, I now understand things better because of my journey. You see this is another reason why I am grateful for my journey and my second chance. People need to love themselves before being able to love others to their full capacity. I am by far not perfect, and it takes two to tango. Thank you for 20 great years Laura.

You too will be a fighter, an advocator, a not sweat the small stuff person, and most of all; you will trust in prayer. Get as many people praying each day or as much as they can. I have seen with my human eyes miracles happen because of thousands using prayer. I am an example.

Also remember how I said that AML M2 is a disease for which you should consider a two steps forward and one step back theory. Well, I was about post 10 months from transplant, and my body was starting to feel terrible. Billy's stem cells and overall blood were in the high 97 to 99% range. Yes, that is right. My blood and cells are 98% my brother Billy, which was picture perfect in that category. What was making me have no energy though? What was causing night sweats? What was the cause of all the weight loss? I went from feeling great to not leaving my bed for over one month.

One night in March 2013, I spiked fever that reached 103.5 degrees. The doctor on call that night at UNC asked me to come to clinic when they opened the next day. He also asked me if I could go to Moore Regional Hospital; although, I already knew that the hospital was at capacity. So I waited until morning, and Jason drove me to UNC. They hit me with a bag of fluids and took cultures out of the port and arm. They hit me with many antibiotics and then many more tests.

I finally received my bed about 10 hours later. Welcome back to 4-Onc. They told me that they had a laundry list of tests lined up over the next four days and to expect a 10 to14-day stay. This was part of the two steps forward and one step back philosophy. Eventually your are going to reach your destination. If you look back at your trek, I know you will recognize the progress.

Long story short, after a lung scope and biopsy, UNC diagnosed me with drug induced toxicity from my anti-rejection medication. My body was so run down that I had temps in the hospital of 105 degrees. Toxicity causes everything that I had been feeling over the previous month and can also cause death if not caught early enough. Of course, I had a couple of bad days during this hospital stay. Nevertheless, my blinds stayed open, I stayed positive, I prayed as I always do, and I trusted my doctors. I received some damage to my lungs, and I needed to take steroids for a few months to correct the damage that the drug gave me. Just a speed bump in my journey. Still making progress though.

UNC also kept me a few extra days to make sure that mold did not show up in my lungs. Mold can be common during the post-transplant 90-day window; however, it is not so common to someone almost 10 months post-transplant. You can get molds anywhere. That is why it is important to wear your mask around large groups of people, especially in closed places such as airplanes. Please make sure you wear your mask every time you are around large groups, on airplanes, and throughout your first year post-transplant. I want to warn you that people will look at you like you have the plague, and you will feel the need to explain to people that you are protecting yourself from them.

Well, my stay consisted of nine days, and I ended up on steroids to build up my lungs. I lost a total of 23 pounds and it sure was going to be great gaining it back. If you have to gain weight back after your transplant please make sure to add whey protein powder to your smoothies. The protein powder will help build your muscles back quicker. Please make sure to get the protein powder approved through your doctor.

So, be ready for the one step back and realize that it is a great time to reconsolidate, refocus, and regroup. You better believe that I visualized being at the beach, fly fishing, watching my boys playing sports, etc. Awe, the love of life. Another quotation to ponder: **"If you love life, don't waste time, for time is what life is made of."** Bruce Lee

I also mentioned in the chapter title that I had a second run-in with my guardian angel. This second run-in included my son Riley. I just purchased Riley a Ford Focus and he had practiced driving for over a one year now. I was still commuting to UNC for bone marrow biopsies and today was the day. We left early in the morning and Riley drove great on the way to UNC. We filled up the car with gas just before we hit Chapel Hill; being that we were ahead of schedule.

The bone marrow biopsy went well, and UNC loaded me up with some meds to comfort me for my ride home. Riley and I were singing to music and having great conversation. The drive from Chapel Hill to Seven Lakes is about an hour and a half and a scenic drive on country roads. Of course, I let Riley drive because he needed the practice. Furthermore, I was loaded up with some sedating medications.

What happened next, just blows my mind to this day. My medications kicked in full-time, and the next thing I knew was that my head leaned up against the passenger side window. I was in a deep sleep almost instantaneously. The issue was that Riley also fell asleep shortly after me. Next, Riley and I are in a snore-off. I am assuming this because we both have the tendency to snore. The car is now easily doing 60 plus MPH on NC15-501. NC 15-501 is a two-lane highway in the country. All of a sudden, I felt bumps and the car was swerving. I remembered the bumps feeling so great; almost like a massage. We woke up and grabbed each other. The car was off of the smooth paved roads and into the highway grass. The highway grass was as tall as the front window; we could not see crap.

This is another reason why I believe in guardian angels and someone is watching over my family and me. Riley grabbed the wheel, as the car was already heading back towards the road. The car was not damaged. Not one speed limit sign hit, not one mailbox hit, not one person or animal hit, and no other cars involved. How does this happen? How did we make it out of this situation unharmed?

Needless to say, Riley is now waiting until 17 to start driving full-time. This was a scene from the movie *Vacation* when *Chevy Chase* is sleeping while driving his family across the country. Thank you Lord and my guardian angels for looking out for us that day. Are you a believer yet? Do you believe in guardian angels yet? Have you experienced such events in your life? I sure do believe in prayer and angels.

As far as my new life—I enjoy going to Brennan's soccer games and Riley's hockey games. I have flown to Florida a few times, with my mask of course, and I have enjoyed seeing family. These are all activities that you must clear through your doctor. Furthermore, you know what you body needs and what your body can handle. My suggestions throughout the book are only suggestions, please be sure to ask your health care professionals and doctors if these are good ideas for you.

My new life post-transplant has also included a trip to Jackson Hole, Wyoming five months post-transplant. Please look at and read the pictures at end of book. I needed to be in Montana and Wyoming again. Man, those trips thrusted new life into me. If you are healthy enough, take advantage of your time before heading back to work. Most allogeneic transplants for AML M2 can take up to two years to fully recover.

Life is great and well worth the bumps and bruises that I have taken to get here. I pray that it will be for you too. As the world turns, I received my immunizations at the one year mark, which was May 14, 2013. Next, I will be heading back to work in August 2013 or when cleared. Life will be normalizing soon; furthermore, I will never go back to my old ways. I will always carry forward my new faith in life and what it has to offer.

I will always help others and stop and smell the roses or great aromas that this world has to offer. Another great benefit that has come of my journey, is that now God puts me into peoples lives that I can help with my knowledge and support. It is as if God has given me a torch to help in lighting up darkness during my travels.

I would like to end this Chapter with a quotation and I hope that this quotation helps you during your trek. The quotation is: **"Life is a gift from the God above. Live each day with peace and love; no matter what storm travels through."** Nishan Panwar

A great quotation that puts life into perspective. The power to do things unimaginable truly comes from within. Remember you have two choices; look at cancer as a gift/opportunity or look at cancer as a burden/ sentence.

This next chapter contains several of my blogs which I typed up on Carepages.com. These blogs are from my actual journey and contain the dates and times they occurred. I hope that you enjoy reading them, and it helps you develop your own blog for your family and friends. There are also more explanations on how the stem cell transplant works and additional quotations to keep you motivated. Enjoy!

CHAPTER 13

EXAMPLES OF MY CAREPAGES/BLOGS

I wanted to keep all of my friends and family in the loop by Carepages. com. Carepages allowed me to update my friends and family on a day-to-day basis. There are also other means that you can use such as: Facebook, CareBridges, Tumblr, Blogger, Blog.com, and Twitter. Typing up my blog each day while in the hospital gave me a sense of accomplishment. It also helped family and friends to not worry as much. They all loved the communication and some people actually became upset if I forgot to post.

My blog gave a quick summarization of how I felt and where my blood levels were on that given day. I gave my weight to show improvements and always included quotations or music links to keep everyone in good spirits.

Here are several of over 200 updates sent, which include quotations, tips, and some stories that were not included in the body of the book:

Lazy Sunday, Answers and Food 4 Thought

Posted Jan 22, 2012 11:52am

Hello All,

I have had some great questions surrounding bone marrow transplant/ stem cell transplant, and the differences between the two options. I have also had questions on what type or subgroup of AML I have? It is to be hoped that I can answer them in this update. In a bone marrow transplant, the donated stem cells are taken from bone marrow. In a stem cell transplant, the donated stem cells are taken from the donors circulating blood.

The choice of which to use depends on many factors, including the type of illness, and the health of the patients own marrow.

How does the donation process work?

—Bone marrow donation is a surgical procedure done in a hospital. The donor is given sedation, and then a needle is used to remove marrow from the hip bones. The donor may have many biopsies performed to give to the needed patient.

—Stem cell donation (peripheral blood) is done in an outpatient setting. The donor is given medication (Neupogen) over several days to increase the number of stem cells in the bloodstream. Then a needle is inserted into an arm vein to draw out blood. The blood passes through a cell separator machine that removes the stem cells. The rest of the blood is returned immediately to the donor. If your cancer is less serious, you may get your own stem cells transplanted. If your blood cancer is serious (AML M2), you will need someone else's healthy stem cells (Allogeneic Stem Cell Transplant). If you receive your own healthy stem cells your comeback is usually less than six months. If you receive someone else's stem cells your comeback can be up to two years because of rejection issues which is called Graft Versus Host disease.

The patient will then stay in the hospital for about 6 weeks for post-transplant care, and usually live within minutes of the transplant facility for 100 days or more while getting post-transplant care.

In some patients, their bone marrow is beyond repair and only a stem cell transplant can offer a cure.

The type of Acute Myelogenous Leukemia I have is AML with maturation or (M2 Subtype). Subtype M2 means that many myeloblasts are present, but some cells are developing toward fully formed blood cells or (mature cancer cells). This is the reason I need a stem cell transplant. My bone marrow is beyond repair and I need to start new with my Brother's stem cells. Once I receive his stem cells, my body will rebuild itself and take on Billy's blood type, etc. Next Billy's stem cells will start creating new WBC's, RBC's and platelets. I will also need all immunizations from birth to 12 years of age before my immune system is fully functional and the transplant is complete. My friend Dan Bruder says it well: "So its analogous to my computer crashing a couple weeks ago and I spent time trying to fix it before wiping it clean and reinstalling all the software and files." Sometimes you just need to wipe your blood and bone marrow clean and start over! I hope that this was helpful in answering some of the questions surrounding my condition.

FOOD 4 THOUGHT (Lazy Sunday Style)

"A Sunday well-spent brings a week of content."
—Old Proverb

"Sunday clears away the rust of the whole week."
—Joseph Addison

"You can't teach people to be lazy—either they have it, or they don't."
—Dagwood Bumstead

Treatment 6 of 10 Today and Food 4 Thought

Posted Feb 18, 2012 2:57pm

Hello All,

So great to hear from my high school and college friends. I hope you all are doing well, and enjoying some of the warm weather we are having :) 62 degrees in Pinehurst today; however, some flurries are scheduled for Sunday evening.

First Health Outpatient Cancer Treatment Center was thoughtful by opening the infusion center for a couple of hours on Saturday and Sunday (this weekend). They did not want me to get admitted into the hospital just to receive my Decitabine. Thank you Tom (Pharmacist), Susan Office Manager, Pat (Transfusion), Bobbie (Nurse), Terri (Nurse), Sandy (Nurse), Barry (Nurse), Lisha (Nurse), Kelly (Nurse), Dr. Moore (Hem/Onc), and Fe (Nurse) for making this happen.

Many people have been asking how I am feeling. Decitabine seems to have less side effects than the last chemo drug. My spine and my bones are hurting—this is because of my numbers are being pulled down. I get tired and I take long naps (yesterday I took a nap from 5:00pm to 9:00pm) and then sleep eight hours at night. I have also had some nausea every day; however, I believe this was from the Duragesic patch (which I pulled off yesterday.)

The great news is that I gained 10 lbs over the last month weighing in at 174 :)) I have been living on Chicken Fajitas :))

FOOD 4 THOUGHT (High School Memories Style)

"True friendship is when two friends can walk in opposite directions, yet remain side by side."
—Author Unknown

"The rain falls regardless if you have a coat or not, but one thing always holds true, someone, somewhere is willing to get soaked with you."
—Author Unknown

"It's our best friends who first teach us how to be selfless—how to give the purest part of ourselves without the expectation of getting anything in return."
—Kierna Mayo

"In the rhythm of life, we sometimes find ourselves out of tune, but as long as there are friends to provide the melody, the music plays on. Thanks for being one of my songs"
—Author Unknown

"There's a big world out there. Bigger than prom, bigger than high school, and it will not matter if you were the prom queen or the quarterback of the football team or the biggest nerd. Find out who you are and try not to be afraid of it."
—Author Unknown

March Madness, Home, and Food 4 Thought

Posted Mar 15, 2012 7:12pm

Hello All,

I hope you are doing well on your brackets for March Madness. For those non-basketball fans; this is the quintessential time for us that like to watch NCAA Basketball. I am eight for eight so far through the round of 64 teams (or 32 games). The little things that makes us HAPPY:))

Dan Grose visited and we had a blast. Laura, Dan, and I picked up where we left off 12 years ago. Unfortunately when we left Florida, we left back a group of great family and friends. Thanks for stopping in Dan:)) You are, and will always be a true friend.

Being home is great! My platelets are 40K, WBC .05 and ANC is .01. All numbers are rising and should double by Monday. Bone marrow is still planned for 21st or 28th of March. I will then start the Decitabine treatments (5 days a month) and then check numbers throughout. One of the benefits of Decitabine is that the patient I will not require many transfusions.

Of course, I am still hoping for the miracle <><. The reality is that I have already failed several of chemotherapies, and it is better for me to start thinking about taking Decitabine for 10 Months. If I get the miracle, then it is icing on the cake and if I do not—then I will not be disappointed. See, it is a win-win situation for me. It will be a miracle if I get to go to transplant or no miracle, and I get to go to a great place also :))))) I hope everyone else sees it that way.

FOOD 4 THOUGHT (College Basketball Style)

"Kids believe practice makes perfect. It doesn't. It makes permanent."
—Mike Jarvis FLORIDA ATLANTIC UNIVERSITY BB COACH, also Boston University, St. John's and George Washington University

"I had a really bad temper, when I was growing up. Sport helped me channel that temper into more positive acts."
—Mike Krzyzewski DUKE

"Most people have the will to win, few have the will to prepare to win."
—Bobby Knight INDIANA UNIVERSITY and Texas Tech

"To me, there are three things we all should do every day. We should do this every day of our lives. Number one is laugh. You should laugh everyday. Number two is think. You should spend some time in thought. Number three is, you should have your emotions moved to tears, could be happiness or joy. Think about it. If you laugh, you think, and you cry, that is a full day. That is a heck of a day. You do that seven days a week, you are going to have something special."
—Jim Valvano NC STATE UNIVERSITY (He lost a 1 Year Cancer Battle)

"A coach is someone who can give correction without causing resentment."
—John Wooden UCLA

"A basketball team is like the five fingers on your hand. If you can get them all together, you have a fist. That is how I want you to play."
—Mike Krzyzewski Duke

Prayers Have Been Answered!

Posted Mar 30, 2012 5:37pm

Happy Friday,

My results came back early and I received my phone call about an hour ago. YOUR PRAYERS WORKED! Thank you for every prayer and every good thought by each of you :)) My blast cells came back at 2% which is classified as remission. I can now continue to stem cell transplant!!!!! The family and I prayed for a clear path or guidance and God answered our prayers. I will be at UNC for four months beginning after the Easter Holiday. I will update you throughout my transplant. God is GREAT!!

Thank you again for all of YOUR LOVE, PRAYERS and SUPPORT!

Love The Hamilton's < > <

A Huge Thank You to Billy!

Posted May 6, 2012 12:20pm

Cheers Everyone,

I hope that this update finds everyone doing well.

Billy has been giving himself four Neupogen shots per day. The Neupogen shots stimulate his stem cells to leave the bone marrow and circulate into his blood. He is flying up today and will spend the day at UNC collecting stem cells on Monday. UNC will freeze his stem cells and transplant them into me on May 14th.

Thank you Billy for being such a wonderful Brother and not thinking twice about giving me a chance of beating AML and MDS.

I love you forever Billy. Thank you from the bottom of my heart :))

We added a photo of the banner that we made Uncle Billy.

___

FOOD 4 THOUGHT (Being Thankful)

"Happiness cannot be traveled to, owned, earned, worn or consumed. Happiness is the spiritual experience of living every minute with love, grace, and gratitude."
—Denis Waitley

"In daily life we must see that it is not happiness that makes us grateful, but gratefulness that makes us happy."
—Brother David Steindl-Rast

"Let us be grateful to people who make us happy;
they are the charming gardeners who make our souls blossom."
—Marcel Proust

Transplant and Update

Posted May 15, 2012 4:22pm

Hey All,

I hope this update finds you enjoying your week. I am sitting next to my wonderful mother Madeleine while typing my update for you. I love you so much Mom!

The transplant went well and even though it was exciting for me, it was like watching paint dry for the nurses and staff. The process entailed 13 tubes of Billy's stem cells; each to be defrosted and pumped into my port. Each tube brought on a surge of energy; a new life:))

The nurses had me suck on peppermints to keep the smell of the chemical down in the room. The chemical is DMSO and is used in the freezing process. Even though I did not taste or smell the DMSO, the nurses and staff said it smells like garlic or creamed corn or tomato soup—great!!!!

The tough part has started today with steroid/chemo pushes. My numbers will plummet down to nothing and it will be a tough two weeks coming up. If you do not hear from me for a few days—please do not worry.

One neat tidbit I forgot to add was that my Late Nana's Birthday was May 14th which made my cell day even more special:))

FOOD 4 THOUGHT

(My Mom's favorite quotation)

"Yesterday is history. Tomorrow is a mystery. Today is a gift, that is why they call it the PRESENT!" Unknown Author

Day 18 Update and Food 4 Thought

Posted May 26, 2012 10:31pm

Hey All,

I hope that everyone is enjoying their Memorial Day Weekend. Laura and the Boys traveled up to Chapel Hill yesterday and stayed overnight. They stayed at the SECU House and traveled back and forth.

Brennan walked some laps with me today. I have walked a total of 418 laps (500 equals a marathon).

I am going to keep this update short because of side effects. Side-effects kicked in two days ago and are right on schedule. Fever was the first sign of issues. I have been flirting with 103 degrees a few times; nevertheless, most of my fevers are low-grade. They now have me on three antibiotics and I will hopefully clear-up soon.

I have also had mouth sores—so bad that I cannot eat. The sores (dime-size) that I have in my throat are inflamed and I look like Stay-Puff Marshmallow Man.

Thanks again for all of your thoughts and prayers.

Food 4 Thought (Hot Summer Days)

"A life without love is like a year without summer."
—Swedish Proverb

"A perfect summer day is when the sun is shining, the breeze is blowing, the birds are singing, and the lawn mower is broken."
—James Dent

"A single sunbeam is enough to drive away many shadows."
—St. Francis of Assisi

Day 19 and Ricky Update

Posted May 27, 2012 9:17pm

Hey All,

Happy Pre-Memorial Day! Please save me a hamburger and a hotdog for when I escape these four walls:))

I forgot to update you on my stats last night and most importantly my friend Ricky. Ricky lost his battle with AML two days ago and his Memorial Services were held today. Please send your prayers out for Joni and Austin tonight—for they are needing comfort through this difficult time. Ricky's cancer came back too strong after his transplant and he had many difficulties with C-Diff, VRE, bacteria in his blood and mold in his sinuses.

I would like to say thank you for letting me know you Ricky. You are a true inspiration to me and I would not be able to do this without your courage to fight AML. I hope you are swinging those golf clubs up in heaven :)

As far as my stats:
Weight 169 Lbs.
WBC .9
ANC .2
HCT 27
PLT 62k
443 Laps completed

It has been two days since I have eaten anything. My mouth, throat and lips are swollen and look like they are sunburnt from the inside out. Feels like another tonsillectomy and I hope now that my numbers are coming back that my pain level will go down. This is all part of the journey and the price that one pays for admission on the transplant ride:))

As far as Food 4 Thought for this update, please help me pray for Ricky's family. Please pray that they find comfort during this time of difficulty. I miss you Ricky!

Day 42 Update

Posted Jun 28, 2012 4:41pm

Cheers All,

I hope everyone is doing well. Before I forget, I would like to wish everyone a great 4th of July.

Hard to believe that it is day 42 already. Only 58 more days in Chapel Hill.

How about the Heat? Great to win another World Championship and add another banner to the arena. It was also great to watch Lebron James win his first ring. Maybe all the haters will leave Lebron alone now!

As far as my health, everything is going well. The only side effects I am still having is Graft Versus Host rashes on my hands, arms, and back. I am also experiencing some neuropathy in my hands and feet as well as some pain in my lungs. The Graft Versus Host rash is welcomed, as long as it goes away sometime soon. All the other side effects are from the high dose chemotherapies I received before my transplant. My lung capacity should slowly comeback to normal.

Adam and I are now going to the UNC Wellness Center to workout a couple of days a week. It is to be hoped that this will get my lungs back to normal quicker. When I get someone to take a picture of Adam I will post on carepages.

My stats are as follows:

WBC 6.9
ANC 5.0
HCT 34.2
PLT 189K
Weight 157

FOOD 4 THOUGHT (NATURE)

"There is pleasure in the pathless woods; There is rapture on the lonely shore; There is society, where none intrudes, by the deep sea and music in its roar: I love not man the less, but Nature more."
—Lord Byron

"I am two with nature."
—Woody Allen

"Wilderness is not a luxury but a necessity of the human spirit."
—Edward Abbey

Day 68 Update, Porsche 911's,
and Music Food 4 Thought

Posted Jul 21, 2012 11:51pm

Cheers All,

I hope everyone is enjoying the summer storms lately.

Adam and I have been talking to many of the nurses and doctors at The Bone Marrow Clinic and our topic of conversation lately has been around music. We have had some great conversation around who the Top 10 guitarists and Top 10 drummers are of our era. Well, I have decided to include my Top 10 below in my Food 4 Thought. Please feel free to write back in your comments who you would add to the list or who you would delete off of the list. I found out that this subject is controversial and most people are passionate about who their favorites are. My focus was the 60's, 70's, 80's and beyond.

I also found out that Billy's cells are getting stronger and are now pushing 99% of my total blood and 97% of my total marrow. UNC is happy with my progress.

Oh yeah, I wanted to let you guys know that I got a wild hair this afternoon and told Adam that I wanted to go to the Porsche dealership and test drive the New 911 Carrera S. I was in luck, they just received a brand new 911 Carrera S loaded (manual shift) and I broke it in today. The sales person was super nice and took me on I-40 and then he pulled over and let me drive on back roads and I-40.

WOW, I have not driven a Porsche 911 since parking cars at the Breakers Hotel in Palm Beach, Florida (1985-86). What a great job that I had in college. I was able to drive the first 959 Slant Nose Porsche that hit North America back in 1986 (came in that day through the Port of Palm Beach) while working a late night shift. We also had access to every sports car under the sun during my two years working there, and the 911 Carrera Turbo stood out head and shoulders against the competition back in the 80's.

Getting back to my test drive today—I think the sales guy was white knuckled for a little bit. I was a bit nervous also, being that the sticker price was 119K. The drive on interstate 40 was most memorable. I was in 4th gear and doing 70 and in a blink of an eye approached 120 MPH. This car does Zero to 60 in 4.1 seconds on this particular model. Well, I wish that it never ended. I guess I can hope to win the lottery and then I will go back and buy that 911 Carrera. Adam and I are going back tomorrow so that he can test drive :))

My numbers are as follows:

WBC 7.4
ANC 3.4
HCT 40.2
PLT 201K
Weight 163

FOOD 4 THOUGHT (MUSIC Top 10 Guitarists and Drummers)

Chris' Top 10 Drummers (In no particular order, except # 1 and # 2)

John Bonham, Led Zeppelin
Neil Peart, Rush
Dave Grohl, Nirvana
Phil Collins, Genesis
Stewart Copeland, The Police
Keith Moon, The Who
Ginger Baker, Cream
Buddy Rich, Played for Nat King Cole, Louis Armstrong and Ella Fitzgerald
Michael Shrieve, Santana
Lars Ulrich, Metallica

Chris' Top 10 Guitarists (In no particular order, except # 1 and # 2)

Jimi Hendrix
Jimmy Page, Led Zeppelin
Chuck Berry
Stevie Ray Vaughan
David Gilmour, Pink Floyd
Jack White, White Stripes
Eddie Van Halen, Van Halen
Eric Clapton
Duane Allman, The Allman Brothers Band
Peter Townshend, The Who

I hope that you found some insight on how to write a blog or maybe you were able to pick up on some good quotations. Either way, I hope that you take the time and type up some form of blog. If you are already on Facebook then that is the route I would take. You can create a public page separate from your personal Facebook. You already have the base of friends and family, etc. This will give you a sense of accomplishment each day and will also pass the time a bit faster while going through the chemotherapy, etc.

I always tried to keep the blog upbeat. No one needs to know how much pain your going through; furthermore, most people reading your blog are battling their own ordeals.

CHAPTER 14

EPILOGUE, TAKEAWAYS, AND PICTURES

"You gain strength, courage and confidence by every experience in which you really stop to look fear in the face." ~Eleanor Roosevelt

Today's date is May 31, 2013, and I am hoping that you gain a couple more tips to get you through your journey.

So, how do you beat the odds and keep the faith? Remember to be your own advocate. Remember to think of cancer not as a sentence or burden, but as a gift or a time to reflect on your life. Remember to eat healthy foods for quick comebacks. If approved, drink milkshakes for quick weight gain.

Remember to always keep your blinds open day and night—you never know what you are going to miss. Remember to include family and friends in your journey. Many people shun their closest of friends and family away because it is easier to not explain the pain. We have the tendency to ball up and keep it all inside us; however, please avoid balling up at all costs.

"Attitude is a little thing that makes a big difference." Winston Churchill

If someone offers you a gift, please accept it with grace. You will most likely have the opportunity to return the favor sometime in life. Remember that prayer, faith, exercise, and meditation in any form your prefer will get you better results every time.

Remember to watch out for elderly drivers, sleepy drivers, and of course young drivers. Explore angels and life after life through reading, especially if you do not believe in such a spiritual universe. Keep in mind that there is always someone else out there that is suffering or hurting more than you. Do not become bitter over your diagnosis, because you have two paths to take with your attitude. Another quotation that may help: **"We cannot change the cards we are dealt, just how we play the hand."** Randy Pausch

Keep in mind that you get a lot more with honey and sugar than you do with vinegar. Remember that this is a journey and not a destination. You can help determine your outcomes through positive mind, exercise, and faith. Remember to visualize what you will be doing when you complete your treatments and get to your cure.

Bear in mind that you will have dark days, and many awesome days. On those dark days keep your chin up and your blinds open. The trek you make will take turns and steps back; however, do not worry because better news is just around the corner. Try to do a blog. You can inspire many people to pull through their personal health issues or personal battles that they may be trying to beat.

Give much attention to your caregivers because they get little credit for what they are achieving. Get outside when possible and when approved by your doctors and nurses. Take vacations between treatments. I am certainly glad I took vacations because six plus months of chemotherapy is a long period without reflecting and enjoying time with your family.

Remember to be your own advocate and demand what you need for your overall good. This is your body, and you know your own body better than any doctor ever will. Write down notes and questions for doctors/nurses, so that you have a clear explanation of what is going on during your treatments and surgeries. Do not be afraid of any doctor. Furthermore, do not feel inferior because doctors put their pants on one leg at a time.

Remember not to sweat the small stuff, because all of that small stuff adds up to a whole lot of unneeded stress. Read books and take advantage of your down-time. Do things that you normally would not have time to do. Take time to tell your kids and family how you feel about them. Tell your kids each day how proud you are of them and how much you love them. Be open with your children and please include them in your journey, depending on age of course. Thank your nurses and healthcare professionals. Many times Laura and I purchased trays of food and placed them back in their break rooms. They loved the food and the attention. Cancer nurses have a tough and emotional job, so be sure to acknowledge them as much possible.

Do not forget to give back or pay it forward to the organizations that helped you along the way. Remember that cancer patients need help to navigate through their journey/battles. This book is also supporting four great causes that help patients financially survive these diagnoses. I heard a great analogy during my long journey and the saying goes like this:

"You cannot take any withdrawals out of life, if you do not make any deposits along the way!" Unknown Author. What a great motto to shape your life. Just think that if everybody lived by this motto—the world would be a much nicer place to live.

Hold on, the book is not over yet. Furthermore, I want to personally thank each of you that purchased this book. I hope that you were able to come away with many ideas that help throughout your life.

May you have many blessed days ahead of you, and may you have the strength and courage to help you through anything that may come your way. May you always remember that **"Beauty is everywhere around us; all you have to do is open your eyes and the possibilities will unfold before you."** Chris J. Hamilton.

I have also included a few pictures of the many nurses and staff that took care of me. You will also see many pictures of my travels post-transplant care. Please read the precautions before you travel and enjoy your journey the best you can.

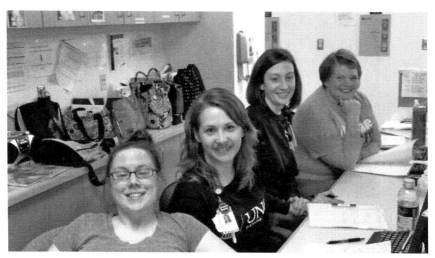

Some of the greats on 4th Floor Oncology. Front to back: Emily, Becca, Claire, and one of my all time favorites Sonja. Nurses that work in Oncology are the hardest working and most giving people you will ever meet. The emotional affect on oncology and hematology nurses is beyond explanation. Thank you for all that you do for each cancer patient. A special thanks to Sonja—you were always a lift to my spirits throughout my stay. I will never forget the good laughs that we shared.

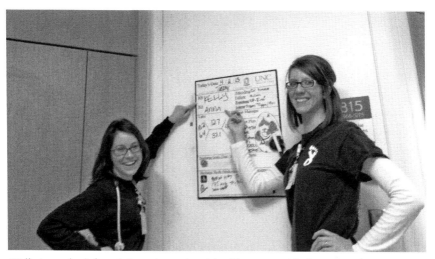

Kelly is on the left and Anna is on the right. Two more 4th floor Oncology greats. I was Kelly's first patient back on 11/11/11. Thank you to all of my great nurses and outstanding care. Thanks goes out to Kelly for doing such an outstanding job. I was also lucky enough to get Kelly again during my nine day hospital stay in April 2013.

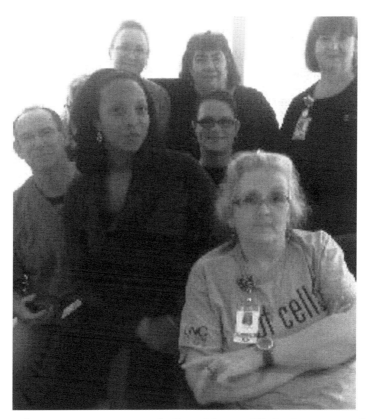

Some of my awesome support at the Bone Marrow Clinic after my transplant. Laura in front, and to the left of her Alicia my P.A., and to the left of Alicia is Andrew, in middle or to right of Andrew is Paula, to right of Paula is Sandra, to left of Sandra is Robin and back left is Ann. You all are awesome people and rightfully deserve to be in the Top 5 Bone Marrow Clinics in the Country (2012). Congratulations on your success and Thank You for you generosity, care, and love.

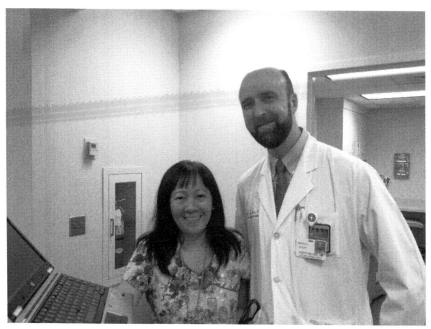

Two of my favorites at First Health Outpatient Cancer Center, Pinehurst. Medical assistant Fe (Left) and Oncologist, Dr. Moore (Right) showed me much love and support during my journey. Dr. Moore and Fe went out of their way to adapt with my schedule at UNC. Dr. Moore always showed optimism and made me feel comfortable. You both are such great people. Thank you Fe, Dr. Moore, and all the special staff of First Health Outpatient Cancer Center. I will never forget that you opened the transfusion center on the weekend, so that I could get my Saturday and Sunday Decitabine chemotherapy treatments. That treatment was one of the *CHE-MOments* that brought me to remission and moved me on to transplant. Thank you so much for your Love and Support. Thank you also to Tom (Pharmacist), Susan Office Manager, Pat (Transfusion), Bobbie (Nurse), Terri (Nurse), Sandy (Nurse), Barry (Nurse), and Kelly (Nurse).

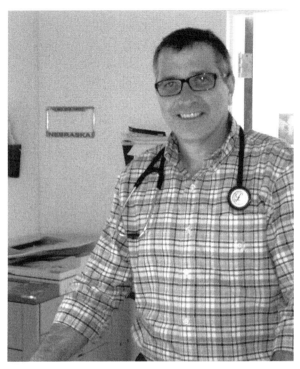

Here is a picture of Dan Matthews, my family physician that has always been there for me. Dan you have always been a great friend, mentor, and one of the best medical practitioners that I have every met. Dan predicted that I had blood cancer even before my first bone marrow biopsy. Thank you for everything Dan.

The next batch of pictures are from post-transplant. Please be sure to check with your doctor before you travel. There are many risks involved with traveling. Nevertheless, I wanted to spend as much time with my family and friends as possible during my first year post-transplant. AML M2 has great success rates with stem cell transplants 6 months out; however, as you get further out, complications can persist with GVHD (Graft Versus Host). It is tough to make it through the first year without a hick-up or two. Remember to always wear your mask while traveling the first year. Be sure to get plenty of rest and do not miss your medications that protect you against viruses, bacteria, etc. Many of the following pictures are from my travels. You have to live life to the fullest. Please take it slow during your comeback. Remember that travel might not be approved for your situation, so please talk to your doctors. Enjoy the pictures.

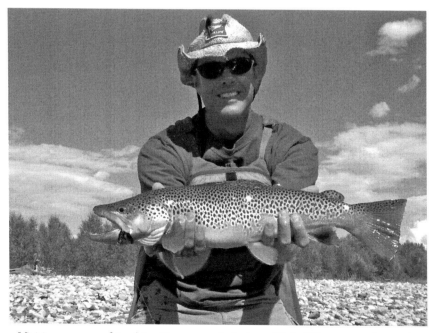

Visiting my great friend Joe Kmetz out in Jackson Hole, Wyoming—5 months after stem cell transplant. Check out that brown trout that Joe caught outside of Bozeman, Montana. Thank you Joe for all the memorable vacations out west over the years. Our memories together at FAU and over the last 25 years are the best.

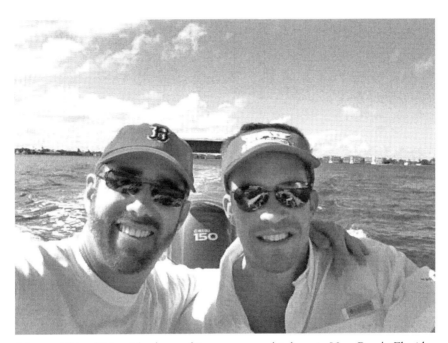

My good friend Marc Tomberg taking me out on his boat in Vero Beach, Florida.
Thank you for your generous friendship over the years Marc. This picture was
taken about 7 months after stem cell transplant. My face and body was a little
puffy from Prograf. Nevertheless, my hair was definitely growing back and had
the consistency of baby hair. We could not stay out long because of the sun.
Prograf and Bactrim have warnings on sun exposure, so please read up and be
careful. Make sure to use heavy sun-block for the rest of your life, because chemo
makes you vulnerable to skin cancer.

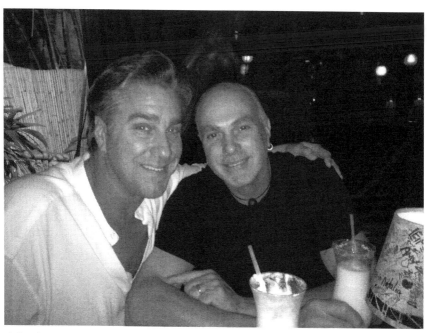

Thank you Joseph Roehm (Billy's partner on right) for holding down the flower shop while Billy was traveling up to UNC Cancer Hospital to deliver his stem cells. Billy and Joseph own one of the BEST flower shops in Delray Beach, Florida. If you are ever in town please stop by "From Roehm With Love." Billy and Joseph fed me for weeks straight to get me back to my fighting weight. Thank you Joseph and Billy for all your spiritual guidance and faith in what miracles God can do.

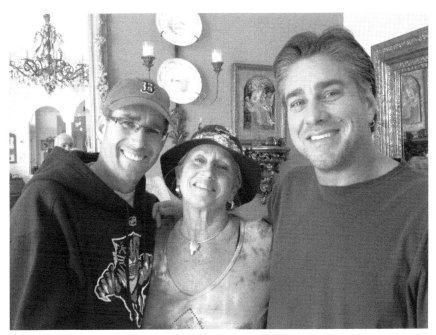

Picture of Mom Hamilton (in Middle) and Billy (to Right) just after a great Thanksgiving meal. Wow, we have so much to be thankful for in life. This picture was taken six months after my transplant. I love you so much Mom and you are not only my Eagle, you are also an angel. I love you more than I can put in words—Thank you!

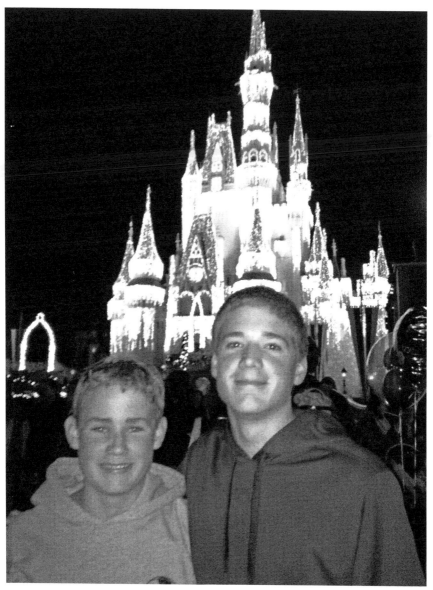

Riley and Brennan enjoying a night at Walt Disney World during Christmas time (seven months after transplant). They had a blast and I wanted to spend as much time with my boys, family, and friends during the first year after transplant. Please include all the family and friends that you can during your journey.

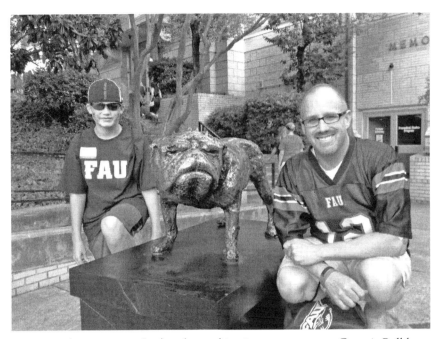

Brennan (my youngest Son) and me taking in a great game at Georgia Bulldog Sanford Stadium (four months after allogeneic stem cell transplant.) My FAU OWLS hung on in a great first half keeping the score within 14 points and then the SEC Bulldog depth kicked in during the second half. Steve and Alex Miller treated Brennan and I, and they drove us to the game. Thank you for your friendship and hospitality Miller's. We especially had a blast at the FAU Alumni Pre-Party. The music and company was so memorable. Thank you FAU Alumni Association. I am proud to be a lifetime Alumni Member of my beloved FAU OWLS. I was nervous being around a large group of people only four months out from transplant. Nevertheless, I survived and enjoyed the game.

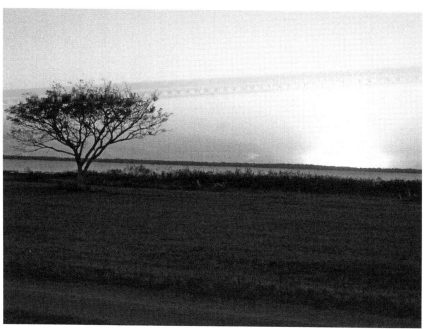

View from Mom and Dad Hamilton's front yard. They have these beautiful sunsets every clear night. Thank you for all the love, great meals, and care during my recovery Mom and Dad. I Love you both to God's house and back!

It is amazing how many people do not stop to enjoy a sunset or sunrise. During my flight down to Florida I was landing in Tampa. I could not believe how beautiful the sunset was from the plane window. This sunset was spectacular and I looked up and back through the plane, and maybe one or two other people were taking in this beautiful site. This plane was packed, and it seemed like every person was on their electronic device. You will notice after your journey that so many things change, and you will truly have a different appreciation for life.

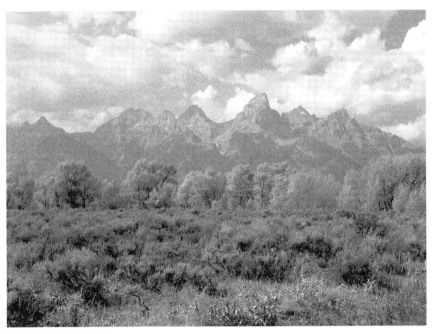

One more picture of Jackson Hole, Wyoming. This is a place that I visualized about during my journey. I needed to see Montana and Wyoming again! If you are feeling well enough, I highly suggest you get out and do it (with the blessing of your doctor.) Positive attitude and willingness to do these activities will help with getting your strength and health back quickly. I wore my mask on all flights, made sure I did not miss any medications, and constantly washed my hands. I stayed healthy throughout my first year, with the exception of a toxicity to one of my medications.

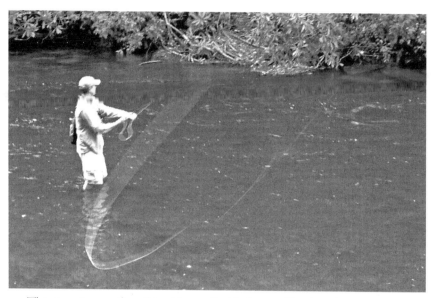

This is a picture of my friend Jason Smith. Jason offered to drive me to the mountains to fly fish with him several times. Unfortunately, I only felt well enough to go on three trips. This particular trip I took pictures while watching Jason fish. The other two trips I was strong enough to fly fish from the shore and catch many trout. Thanks again for your friendship Jason. Also, thank you for being my second pair of eyes reading the book, and for your creativity working with the title.

The next two pictures are of my transplant doctor and my transplant coordinator at UNC Cancer Hospital. Dr. Serody (pictured below) is my "triple threat." The reason why I call him this, is because he has been trained in Hematology, Immunology, and Microbiology. He is brilliant, and I was lucky to get him as my stem cell transplant doctor. Thank you for putting up with me Dr. Serody, and for making sure that I stayed healthy throughout my transplant. I was nervous during my transplant and you definitely put me at ease.

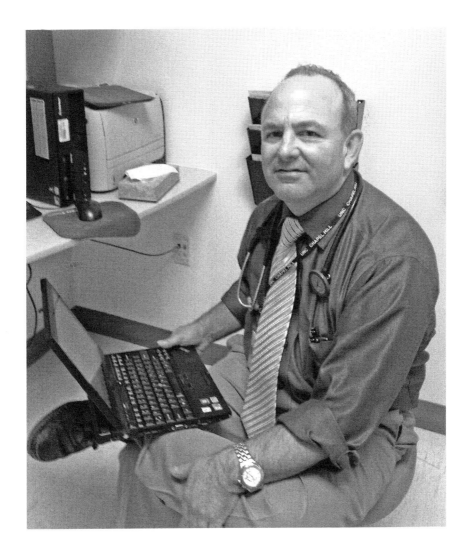

Below is a picture of a special person that absolutely loves her job at UNC. Debbie coordinates every stem cell transplant patient and their donor. The process can take several months from when the patient is diagnosed and all the way through to transplant. I have no idea how she does it at all. Debbie, thank you for working so hard to get me to transplant. Definitely the best decision I have made during my two year journey. Please know that the knowledge of your team made my decision that much easier. A special thanks goes out to Alicia (Billy's coordinator).

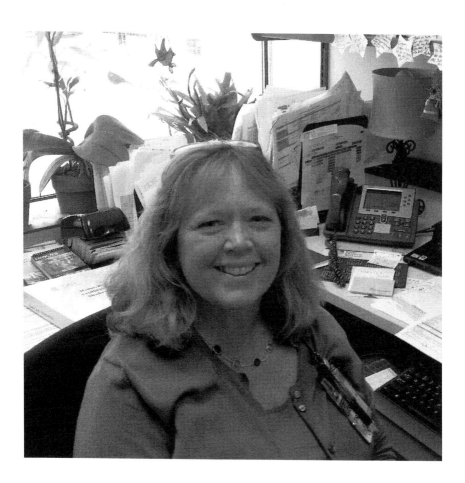

DEFINITIONS AND MEDICAL TERMINOLOGY SECTION

Aciphex—Also known as Rabeprazole is an anti-ulcer drug or a proton pump inhibitor medication used in reducing acid in the stomach.

Actigall—Also known as Ursodiol. Is a Medication used to protect the liver and can aid in dissolving gall stones.

Allogeneic Stem Cell Transplant—Patient receives blood forming stem cells or peripheral blood stem cells from another healthy person such as a sibling or unrelated donor. Once the cancer patient receives high-dose radiation/chemotherapy, the healthy stem cells are then transplanted into the patient.

AML—Acute Myelogenous Leukemia, also known as Acute Myeloid Leukemia is an aggressive cancer of the blood cells and bone marrow. Most cases of AML will require a stem cell transplant for a possible cure or remission.

ANC—Absolute Neutrophil Count is a measure of the number of neutrophils present in your blood.

Antidepressant—Medication that treats depression.

Anti-fungal—A drug used for treating and preventing fungal infections. Fluconazole is the drug of choice in cancer clinics.

Anti-Rejection Medication—Also called immunosuppressants. This medication helps to suppress the body's immune system response to a new organ. Helps the body to not reject new organ or stem cells.

Antiviral—A drug used to treat and prevent viral infections. Valtrex is the drug of choice in most cancer hospitals.

Aphaeresis Machine—Medical machine in which blood of a donor or patient is passed through an apparatus that separates out stem cells and returns the remainder of blood back into circulation.

Ativan—Also known as Lorazepam. Is a medication used to treat anxiety disorders and can also be utilized to treat insomnia.

Autologous transplant—A transplant procedure removing and reserving the patient's own stem cells. Next they treat the patient with high dose chemotherapy and radiation to kill the cancer cells. Once the patient is treated, they transplant the good stem cells back into the patient through transfusion.

Bone Marrow—The vascular tissue within the bone that contains red blood cells, white blood cells, and stem cells.

Bone Marrow Biopsy—A biopsy that is utilized to evaluate the bone marrow and health of the patient's white blood cells, red blood cells, and platelets. A local anesthetic is used to numb the patient's back bone located above their buttocks. Next, a needle will be inserted into the patient's bone to collect a liquid sample of blood and marrow.

Carcinoma—Most common form of cancer that usually starts in the tissue lining of the body or the epithelial tissue of the skin.

Chemo or Chemotherapy—is the treatment of cancer with cytotoxic antineoplastic drugs that work to kill the intended cancer or disease.

C-diff—Also known as Clostridium Difficile. C-Diff is a bacteria and can cause severe diarrhea and other intestinal issues when it takes over the good intestinal gut flora.

Creatinine Clearance—the rate at which waste or creatine is cleared from the blood through the kidneys.

Cytogenetics—The study of chromosomes and cells. Hematologists utilized a test to evaluate the health of your chromosomes or cells in your bone marrow.

Decitabine—Also known as Dacogen. A drug that is used for the treatment of Acute Myeloid Leukemia (AML) and Myelodysplastic Syndromes (MDS). Decitabine is in a class of medications called hypomethylation agents.

Diflucan—Also known as Fluconazole. Diflucan is an Anti-fungal drug used to treat the prevention of superficial and systemic fungal infections.

D.M.S.O.—Stands for Dimethyl Sulfoxide and is a colorless liquid. The solvent is used in many medications to penetrate the skin and help with drug delivery. D.M.S.O. is also utilized in the freezing process of the stem cells.

Engraftment—Engraftment is when transplanted stem cells start to grow in the bone marrow of the recipient and begins to produce healthy white blood cells, red blood cells, and platelets.

E.N.T.—Stands for Ear, Nose and Throat Doctor or otorhinolaryngologist who specializes in the treatment of head and neck disorders.

Exalgo—Also known as Hydromorphone Hydrochloride. Exalgo is a mu-opioid agonist and is used in the treatment of moderate to severe chronic pain.

Follicular Papillary Carcinoma—The second most common type of thyroid cancer. These cancers are usually found as a lump/nodule on or within your thyroid gland.

Grand Rounds—A formal clinical gathering usually at the beside of the patient. Also known as making rounds. Grand rounds are common practice at teaching hospitals.

G.V.H.—Stands for Graft Versus Host Disease. G.V.H. is a common problem following a organ, tissue, or stem cell transplant. Doctors use anti-rejection medications to keep G.V.H. at bay. The most common affected areas of GVH are the skin, stomach, intestines, liver, and possibly lungs.

GY—Gray unit of absorbed radiation to the tissue or body.

Hematologist—A hematologist is a specialist that studies blood disorders, such as leukemia, lymphoma, and anemia.

Hemoglobin—A protein that is responsible for transporting oxygen in the blood. Hematologists measure hemoglobin to diagnose anemia.

Hypothyroidism—Is a condition when the thyroid gland is not producing enough thyroid hormone. A low level of thyroid hormone makes you feel tired and weak.

Incentive Spirometer—Otherwise known as a spirometer. This is an instrument that measures the amount of air that travels to and from the lungs. Also is a small device which is used to strengthen the lungs.

Intramuscular—This medical term is utilized to describe the location of an injection site into the a muscle.

HCT or Hematocrit—The percentage or ratio of red blood cells to your total blood.

Leukemia—A type of blood or bone marrow cancer which is a result of an abnormal increase of immature white blood cells. Heath care professionals refer to the immature WBC's as blasts.

Levaquin—Also known as Levofloxacin. Levaquin is an antibiotic from the class of fluoroquinolones. Levaquin is used to treat bacterial infections of the sinuses, skin, kidneys, lungs, bladder, or prostate.

Liver Function Tests—(LFT or LF) A group of blood tests that detect inflammation or damage to the liver.

M2—Stands for a subtype of AML or Acute Myeloid Leukemia also known as AML with maturation.

MDS—Stands for Myelodyspastic Syndrome (pre-leukemia). A disease that affects the bone marrow and blood cells. Can be mild to severe, and if not treated in time can turn into leukemia.

Millicurie—A unit of radiation used in measuring nuclear medicine.

Meditation—Is the practice or art of training your mind to enter a state of relaxation by focusing on one's thoughts.

MRSA—Stands for Methicillin-resistant Staphylococcus Aureus (MRSA) and is a type of staph bacteria that is resistant to most antibiotics.

Mucositis—Inflammation and irritation of the gastrointestinal tract. Mouth sores and extreme pain are common with mucositis.

Narcotic—Is a type of pain killer utilized for treating moderate to severe pain.

NSAID—Stands for Non-Steroidal Anti-inflammatory Drugs. They are among the most common pain relief medicines available for prescription and over-the-counter. An example would be Ibuprofen or Aspirin.

Norvasc—Also known as amlodipine besylate. This blood pressure medicine belongs to a group of drugs called calcium channel blockers or vasodilators. Norvasc works to relax blood vessels thereby decreasing blood pressure.

Nuclear Medicine—The use of radioactive substances for the treatment of cancer cells or disease.

Neupogen—Also known as filgrastim or GCSF (granulocyte colony-stimulating factor.) Is a drug utilized to treat neutropenia or low white blood cells. Can also be utilized to force stem cells into a patients blood circulation.

Neutropenia—Also known as leukopenia. This term is used when a patients white blood cell count is low or below normal and puts the patient at risk of infection.

Obama Care—Also known as The Patient Protection and Affordable Care Act or healthcare reform. Most of the reform, laws and taxes go into effect in 2014.

Oncologist—Medical professional that specializes in treating cancer.

PA-C or PA—Stands for Physicians Assistant that is trained to practice medicine under a supervision of a doctor.

PENNSAID—Is a topical non-steroidal anti-inflammatory drug (NSAID) used for treating the signs and symptoms of osteoarthritis of the knee or knees. This medication contains D.M.S.O. to aid with penetration of the skin.

Platelets—They are the clotting cells of the blood. A normal platelet count is 150,000 to 450,000. You have to receive a platelet transfusion when your platelets drop below 10,000.

Port for Chemo—Is a small device that is implanted underneath your skin and is used to draw blood or infuse chemotherapy.

Port Needles—Needles that allow nurses to access your port underneath your skin. The needles can stay in for up to one week. The needles are used to deliver medications and chemotherapy to the patient.

Post-Transplant Care—Means medical care after a transplant. Usually consists of 100 Days following an Allogeneic stem cell transplant. The immunosuppressed patient requires specialized care sometimes daily.

Prograf—Otherwise known as Tacrolimus. Prograf weakens your body's immune system, thereby, preventing the destruction of the newly transplanted organ or stem cells.

RBC or Red Blood Cells—Mature blood cells that carry oxygen from the lungs to tissues throughout the entire body.

Radiologist Oncologist—Is a medical doctor that specializes in the treatment of cancer using radiation.

Remission—Complete or temporary eradication of the signs and or symptoms of cancer.

Stem Cells—Are (mother cells) that create new white blood cells, red blood cells, and platelets.

Sterilize—Is a process of disaffecting and eliminating disease causing micro-organisms.

Streptococcus Pneumoniae—Is a gram positive bacteria that can enter through your upper respiratory tract. The bacteria can cause pneumonia, sinusitis, meningitis, and otitis media—just to name a few.

Squamous Cell Carcinoma—Cancer of the epithelial or squamous cells. These cells or cancer are found on skin, inside the mouth, or in the throat.

Thyroid—One of the largest glands in the human body located in the lower neck area. The thyroid gland controls your metabolism which determines how quickly your body uses energy.

Tonsillectomy—A procedure that an Ear, Nose, and Throat doctor utilizes to remove the tonsils—mainly in children due to chronic infections.

Ultram—Also known as Tramadol. Ultram is a centrally-acting analgesic that treats moderate to moderately sever pain.

Vancomycin—A strong antibiotic utilized to treat resistant bacteria.

VRE—Stands for Vancomycin Resistant Enterococcus and are bacteria called enterococci that develop resistance to many antibiotics. Cancer patients can develop severe diarrhea from VRE due to their weakened immune system.

White Blood Cells—Also known as leukocytes. WBC's are the infection fighting blood cells, which protect patients against infections and disease.

Zofran—Also known as Ondansetron. This medication is utilized to prevent nausea and vomiting induced by chemotherapy, radiation, and surgery. Drug of choice for Oncology/Hematology patients that experience nausea during chemotherapy.

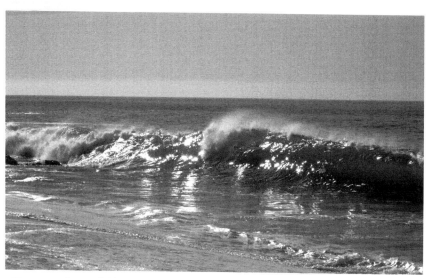

One more beautiful beach picture to help you with relaxation. Cabo San Lucas, Mexico. This picture is also a tribute to my Aunt Yvonne's poem on the next page.

A POEM THAT AUNT YVONNE WROTE

FOR ME DURING MY BATTLE/JOURNEY

Chris' fight with cancer like troubled waters, using this analogy because he loves surfing!!

Troubled waters seem to flow
Creating havoc wherever they go
Bearing matters of debris
Strong winds whipping up the seas

Trying times to ride the waves
Not bringing on the raves
From those trying to reach the shores
Like opening up some safety door

Tidal waves, howling winds
Shrieking as if it sings
Life being raked across the coals
Causing pain, penetrating our souls

Families of those thought lost at sea
Standing hopeful along with me
Together, praying for those we love
As the sea continues to rise above the bluff

Suddenly, a peace comes with each wave
The ocean no longer their grave. A break in treatment
Their souls now back home with thee
Together, awaiting no longer at sea

In life always in our mind and heart
Awaiting the next troubled waters to start
For our life is full of strife to greet
All our fate to face indeed

Love, Aunt Yvonne

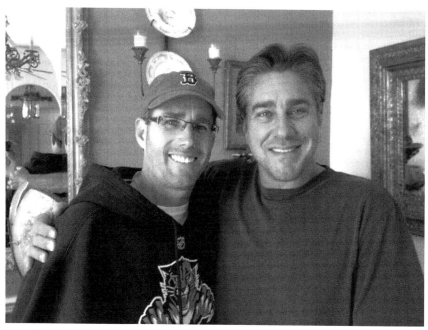

Another awesome photo of my brother Billy. I cannot thank you enough. I am so glad that I was able to take this journey with you. Our pilgrimage over the last two years has brought us closer together, and has opened my eyes on how important family is in this world. Thank you for saving my life Billy. I love you forever!!!!!